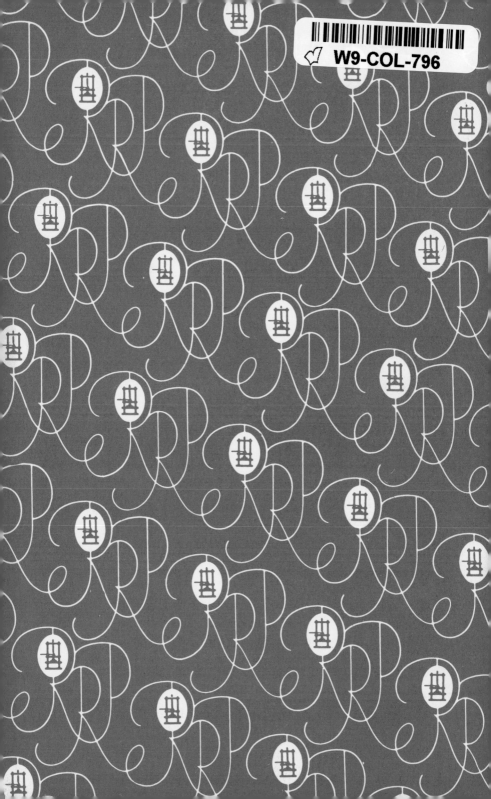

EXCELLING
THE NUTRITIONAL WAY TO GOOD HEALTH

Excelling

THE NUTRITIONAL WAY TO GOOD HEALTH

by Cecilia Maguire

THE ROSEN PUBLISHING GROUP

New York

Published in 1985 by The Rosen Publishing Group, Inc.
29 East 21st Street, New York, N.Y. 10010

First Edition

Library of Congress Cataloging in Publication Data

Maguire, Cecilia.
    Excelling the nutritional way to good health.

    1. Youth—Health and hygiene. 2. Nutrition.
3. Food, Junk. I. Title.
RA777.M25   1985   613'.0433   85–1724
ISBN 0–8239–0635–3

Manufactured in the United States of America

About the Author

Cecilia Maguire is a free-lance writer in the scientific and health fields who has contributed chapters on those areas to a number of books and several national magazines. She has researched and ghost-written four books on medicine and health guidance for vascular surgeons. Having worked as a daily newspaper reporter after undergraduate school, later while in graduate studies at New York University she worked with young adults and law students of the Western Hemisphere. Her interest in young-adult health and nutrition was heightened while she was employed in public relations and writing for the U.S. Public Health Service in Washington, D.C. and as a writer for the (then) National Tuberculosis Association in New York. Young people were also targets for her writing while working in public relations for Town Hall and the Lincoln Center for the Performing Arts in New York.

Contents

Introduction

Most of us marking birthdays in the teens—the truth is we're really young adults—at times can really feel persecuted by spurts of parent "advice." That so-called advice really takes the form of criticism, which more often than not has the tag line "for your own good."

A lot of it has to do with turn-off topics like a chronically messy room, your taste (and volume) in record albums, better homework habits, or less TV watching.

One of the worst drags of all times has been the static about most of your favorite foods: "That junk is going to ruin your stomach!" "Stop snacking and leave room for real food!" "That stuff is going to ruin your complexion (or teeth)!"

Know what? Those parents and teachers could have the right message about what you should be eating, or not eating, even though they are not a cool under-thirty. Besides being older and more experienced, they are more likely to digest newspaper and magazine articles with the right dope on nutrition. They are really concerned because they know that these are extra-important years when it comes to building your bodies and fighting disease and infection. They want to pass what they have learned on to you at a critical time. You can't blame them.

Maybe we're all getting more flak these days on eating and food because nutrition is really a young science that seems to pose more questions than it can come up with answers. In spite of so-called advances in nourishment knowledge, we've added little in the last century to info on just how food-fuel feeds our bodies.

We *all* have a lot to learn about the scene—including the doctor, the food specialist, the nutritionist, and whoever else is professionally and practically involved in this infant profession.

What Is "Food," Anyhow?

Food is a form of fuel, not for the family car or the furnace, but for the human body. We get a lot of heavy messages these days about "fuel shortages" and "the high cost of energy." But those refer mostly to "fossil fuels," preserved animal or plant remains from past ages that we mine out of the earth to produce heat or power or both. Whether we eat our food for fuel or pay for the other kind of fuel, the result is virtually the same. As a matter of fact, in some cases *fuel* has become a synonym for *nutrient*, whether for plant, animal, or human body.

Then what is a nutrient? A nutrient is something that nourishes, feeds, supports, makes repairs, supplies energy, causes to grow and develop. In that respect, food and its nutrients are far superior to what goes into the gas tank of the family car. The best and most expensive brand of unleaded gas won't repair the car or supply growth and development. It just makes the car run, temporarily.

About food itself. Fortunately, most of us in this country have plenty of it. (Unfortunately, almost every young American has viewed on TV news or in magazine pictures the swollen bellies and sharply outlined ribs of little children suffering from starvation in other lands.)

Let's go back to high school freshman biology. From stem to stern, or head to toe, our bodies are composed of cells of differing kinds and shapes; you'll remember that a cell is the tiniest basic unit of which any living thing is composed. It's so small that you can see it only with a microscope. The magnifying microscope will show in general the cell's three main living parts: the nucleus (core or center), the cytoplasm (jellylike substance surrounding the nucleus), and the cell membrane (the edge).

Your life started way back because two cells got together in your mother's uterus. From those two cells others multiplied as you grew and developed. Then you developed as an embryo and later a fetus up to the time of your birth.

The cells have tiny powerhouses called *mitochondria* (some individual cells have about 500) that change the food you eat into energy. Cells work hard all the time; they wear out and break down and must be constantly replaced by new ones.

The Food Factory

Your body cannot use the food as it is received via the mouth. The food must be broken down into forms or compounds that the body can use.

You might say that one single morsel of food eaten is acted on by every physiological part of the mouth (teeth, tongue, salivary glands) and then travels down the length of the "conversion plant" by way of departments with specific functions such as esophagus, stomach, small and large intestines, and eventually rectum and anus.

Take a bite of anything—apple, pizza, candy bar—and as you chew it into pulp, saliva from the glands in your mouth helps to soften it. Your mouth and teeth act like the blender in your mom's kitchen. At the same time, an enzyme (chemical reactor) called *ptyalin* changes the sugar in the food into starch.

As you swallow the food, it passes down your esophagus into your stomach, which is like an elastic sac and adjusts its shape to hold however much you may eat.

Muscles of the stomach wall toss and turn the food as it mixes with other body-manufactured chemicals. The busy digestive system needs more help in breaking down the protein in the food you've eaten, and so various enzymes are shot into the process.

An enzyme—called a catalyst or modifier by nutritionists—is a substance made by living tissue that speeds certain chemical changes; we can consider enzymes the body's chemical change-makers. The enzymes are the key to the digestive process. To enable the body to use food-nutrients more efficiently, the enzymes change carbohydrates into simple sugars, proteins into amino acids (organic compounds that are vital to life), and fats into fatty acids and glycerol (a sweet, colorless syrup). Surprisingly, despite the work they do, enzymes aren't used up, but stay intact for future use.

As the food is digested, it is swallowed up in turn by the wall of the small intestine and is siphoned into nearby capillaries (tiny blood vessels); nutrients can be used by the body only after they have entered the bloodstream. The capillaries' blood then conveys the nutrient to the liver; part of the sugar in the blood is converted into animal starch called *glycogen*, which is then stored in the liver for use when needed.

The Lively Liver

Just as the enzyme is the key to the process of breaking down food nutrients for bodily use, the liver is a key to opening the gates to this important process. The liver, the largest organ (except for the skin) of the human body, is one of its most fascinating. It serves as a waste disposal unit as well as an energy storehouse and is charged with no fewer than 500 separate and important tasks. No wonder the whole body is in big trouble when something goes wrong with the liver and its functioning.

Some of the nutrients move into the liver's spongy tissue from the intestines, others from the lymphatic glands. Liver cells are arranged in groups called *lobules*, each of which is about 1/25 of an inch in diameter; and each lobule gets its nutritious blood from the *portal vein*, which connects the liver with the intestines. When it reaches the lobule, the vein branches out to connect with tiny channels called *sinusoids*, which are responsible for transporting the blood to each cell for nourishment.

These cells remove any poisonous substances from the

blood, and they also take a percentage of nutrients to hold for use on demand; 95 percent of the body's intake of vitamin A is stored in liver cells. When that stockpiling is completed, leftover nutrients are carried to a central vein, which transports them to the heart, and that vital organ sets up their distribution throughout the body.

Nutrients that have traveled from liver to heart cross over to the lungs for fresh oxygen, then go back to the heart and are jetted into the aorta, the largest artery of the body, which springs up and arches over from the top of the heart.

Contrasting in size with the aorta, a giant among blood vessels, are the tiny capillaries that supply the head-to-toe arterial route for the nutrients in supplying nourishment.

The Cool Capillary

The average capillary is 7/10,000 of an inch in diameter, which is about 1/5 the diameter of a hair. In some cases, a hair from your scalp is huge in comparison with a capillary. Capillaries are so tiny that blood cells can ooze through them only in single file and very slowly; it is estimated that it can take over two hours for 1/100 ounce of blood to squeeze through the length of one capillary.

How, then, can we say that all the blood in the body can be moved through the hairlike capillary system in a few minutes? Well, there are innumerable capillaries in the body, over 60,000 miles of them—almost three times the length of the United States coastline. And, in good health, the capillaries' performance is cool.

While the blood is oozing through the capillary system, it slips oxygen and nourishing molecules (miniscule compounds) to the cells; at the same time, cell wastes are carried off. The nutrients and discarded wastes squeeze through the barrier in a kind of osmosis (diffusion), past infinitesimal openings through which they are propelled by other molecules pushing behind them. The process works so well that about 90 percent of the time molecules transported by the blood are dropped into the body cells during one trip through the capillary system.

Explaining Elimination

The body's system of elimination is an intricate method of getting rid of the wastes from the foods you eat and the liquids you drink after the body has taken all it can use from them. The elimination process needs a little help in disposing of the wastes from foods. That's why the doctor underlines the need for plenty of water and fiber or "roughage" in your daily diet. Among other benefits, adequate liquid and food fiber are the best encouragements for the body to get rid of poisons and wastes.

For liquid extras that must be discarded, we have two bean-shaped, red-brown organs called kidneys, one on each side of the spine in the "small of the back." In the average young adult, each kidney is about four inches long and two inches wide. The kidneys carry on quite an operation. They are set up (and act) like the best water-filtering plant in your county, but what they filter (strain or purify) is blood. They take waste materials and other toxins from the blood and help equalize and balance its water content with other substances.

Another organ involved in elimination is the bladder. The bladder takes in urine, which is liquid material to be discarded, swelling like a balloon to hold it. It is all literally washed away in urination.

Another way in which the body discards liquid waste is by perspiration or sweat. Although this happens in various ways (even while you sleep), you probably notice it most in the gym or on the tennis court, because sweat production increases with strenuous exercise. In a sense, because it covers every area of your body, the skin is considered the most active and largest organ of the body.

The sweat glands are just beneath the surface of the skin,

where they are surrounded by tiny capillaries. The walls of the capillaries and the sweat glands permit the surplus water and impurities to exchange places, crossing back and forth. When the waste liquid gets into the sweat glands, it is thrown off through the pores (tiny openings) of the skin. You throw off about two pints of water daily by perspiration, four pints or more if the weather is very hot or if you are working out in the gym, bicycling, skating, or running.

Perspiration, besides supplying the makers of deodorants with an exaggerated villain, has another vital use. It helps to regulate the body temperature, as a thermostat controls the heat or air conditioning in your home. It's important to keep the internal organs surrounded by a reasonable temperature. For example, when you exercise your body burns up food more rapidly, as if you were stoking a furnace, and so the body's heat soars. The sweat that forms on the skin evaporates fast and in so doing cools the body to a desirable temperature.

The lungs also throw off excess liquid, about a pint a day, with the carbon dioxide they expel. You've seen people blow on their eyeglasses to get a little moisture on them to clean them. Or you can see the moisture on your breath on a cold day.

Why the Physiology?

We've presented a brief review of elementary or high school physiology to sketch the route and the way in which food, wonderful food, plays a leading role in keeping us alive and well.

We had several good reasons. Maybe, we felt, if we set it down in some detail it might help you realize why parents and teachers seem to sound off so often about "eating right."

Trust us, the human body is a wonderful but intricate machine, one that grows, develops, builds, works, plays, and stays alive mainly on the amount and kinds of food you eat.

The average young adult is not overly concerned with motives such as sound health and long life. But serious surveys and studies have shown that he or she is very much interested in physical appearance, in attracting the opposite sex, in being reasonably confident of dates for school dances, the disco, or sports events.

How might these goals be realized? Good food and balanced meals can't provide the whole answer. Other factors also work toward helping us look more attractive, for example, personal hygiene and neat (not necessarily expensive) clothing.

But look at it this way. A bad diet chock full of empty calories can make you fat and lumpy, particularly if you neglect exercise. If your diet lacks certain vitamins and calcium, your teeth can decay, and you'll lose them at an early age, despite many painful hours with the dentist. Neglecting other basic nourishment can mean ratty hair and dull lifeless eyes; you can even jeopardize your eyesight.

On the other hand, normal conditions and a truly nourishing diet can result in a good physique, clear skin, and shining eyes and hair. Exercise calls for a hefty supply of energy. And where does the energy come from, mostly? Not from some "Star Wars" magic gun. It comes from food, good, nourishing food.

This book will try to interest you in other nonmagic formulas for warding off the ravages of age for as long as possible, avoiding premature lines and wrinkles, heart attack and heart disease. All with the simple aid of the right food.

EXCELLING
THE NUTRITIONAL WAY TO GOOD HEALTH

The Facts:
Food-fuel and Its Fate

It's a safe bet you've heard the comparison, over and over, that your body and the food it takes in are like the run-of-the-mill vehicle and its fuel: family car, bus, motor bike. The engine is there in each, but getting the machine going depends on the fuel—gasoline, battery, whatever. Your body as a human engine depends on *its* fuel—food. The food or fuel is taken in, chewed, broken down into components that the body can use, and off you go.

There's a big difference in the comparison. Your human engine uses its fuel to maintain life, to keep up the critical flow of blood through your body, to help you walk and dance and study, to build more cells for physical growth from infancy to toddler, to preteens, to young adult and later. Your car or bike doesn't build new cells to take the place of worn-out ones; with time and use, it simply wears out.

The food itself is made up of several kinds of substances called *nutrients*. In turn, to break down the food for proper use by all of the body's cells, there is a complex group of parts working like a unit called the *digestive system*. The two major parts of that system are the *alimentary* (nutritive) *canal* and the *digestive glands*.

The alimentary canal is the path or tube through which the food first passes. The digestive glands are special cells or groups of cells that store up and deposit the necessary juices to aid in the digestive process.

The route of the alimentary canal begins with the mouth, followed by the throat, the esophagus or gullet, the small intestine, and the large intestine. The digestive glands, following the same route, are the salivary (mouth) glands, the gastric (stomach) glands, the glands of the pancreas (which secrete digestive juices), and the small and large intestines. The intestines are coiled lengths of tubes that form parts of the canal; *small* and *large* describe the width of the coil, not the length.

Access to the canal is the mouth, where the teeth, tongue, and saliva glands, working together, start the digestive process. First the teeth grind the food into small pieces. The surface of the tongue has *taste buds*, that enable you to experience four kinds of taste: sweet, sour, salty, and bitter. The muscles of the tongue move the food from side to side in the mouth and help the throat muscles in the swallowing process.

After the food slides down the throat, it empties into the stomach, a sac shaped like a "J." The stomach wall has three sets of muscles, which churn the food, mix it with the stomach juices, and propel it into the small intestine, the next stage of its journey.

As the food empties from the stomach into the small intestine, a small valvelike muscle of the lower end of the stomach closes, preventing partly digested food from flowing back into the stomach. The partly digested food contains certain nutrients made up of compounds that cannot directly enter the cells. When these have been digested, they become *end products*, or simpler compounds, which are liquefied and deposited in the lower part of the small intestine. Now made simpler, these compounds can pass through the membranes, or thin covering layers of the cells. The cells can now use the end products to best advantage.

The undigested matter and the water from the food now move from the small intestine to the large intestine, or colon. As the wavy muscular movement called *peristalsis* moves the undigested fluid mass along the large intestine, the linings of the intestine absorb the water and some of the minerals from it. The absorbed substances then go into the bloodstream. The peristalsis process moves the remaining mass (solid waste) to the lower end of the large intestine and then to the rectum.

The solid wastes are stored in the rectum, usually for a few hours, until they are discharged from the body through the anus, an opening located between the buttocks.

The total of all those processes by which the body changes raw material (food, water, oxygen) into cell tissue and energy is called *metabolism*. It is actually a series of chemical changes that use up and release energy.

We hear and read a lot these days about the "balanced diet." What does it all mean? "Balance" in this context means the right amounts of the right foods in the daily diet to promote and maintain health, vigor, and general well-being. Simply, it's eating what and as much as you should.

Throughout your life your cells and tissues (groups of cells) and all your organs depend on food for the wherewithal to repair and rebuild themselves as they wear out or are injured in any way.

It's no small matter of one or two or three types of foodstuffs that can satisfy the need. Nutritional science has just about proved that as many as fifty separate substances among these nutrients are necessary to maintain our lives and our health.

Baby's Building Blocks

Your young-adult food favorites and habits were not formed recently in the fast-food hangout, the supermarket, or the school cafeteria. Those habits (maybe for life) began in infancy. By the time you ordered your first lunch in the high school cafeteria, it may have been too late to change them.

We have seen that the body grows and develops on the food taken into its cells. (The human body, it is estimated, contains more than 50 billion cells). Your mother and her doctor started the whole process five or six months before you were born. Your nourishment first came by way of her body even before she discovered she was pregnant. Thereafter she visited the doctor regularly for prenatal care.

This "pregnancy" was not too much different from her needs when she wasn't carrying a child, but the health habits now concerned, not one, but two people.

The doctor told your mother to get plenty of exercise (not strenuous or exhausting) in the fresh air, plenty of sleep, and rest. Maybe most important of all, the doctor pointed out that a balanced diet of good food was healthful and nourishing to both of you. (Inadequate and junk foods meant *you* would be undernourished in her womb; *she* would become fat or frail, strain her heart and cardiovascular system, and make your delivery difficult.) To protect you and your nourishment, as well as hers, on each visit the doctor checked her blood pressure, urine, kidney function, and water retention.

4

Once you were born, you and your food were almost on your own except for the way you were nourished in the early months. Some of you were nursed (fed at the breast) by your mother; many doctors still call breast milk the "perfect food" for the infant. Others of you had infant formulas. Later came strained fruits and vegetables and liquefied meats.

Let's now discuss a really bad scene called child abuse. For some of us, that phrase evokes pictures of a child beaten unmercifully with a strap or chain, locked in a dark closet, tied to a bedpost, burned with lighted cigarettes. That's the bizarre version.

Some other parents, often without meaning to, practice "nutritional child abuse." Starving their kids? No way, on the surface. Some are plain ignorant or lazy or just don't care what their youngsters are stuffing into their bodies. Instead of a little inconvenient discipline when a kid acts up, they rely upon triple-type "tranquilizers" and outright bribes: candy, cookies, and just plain junk. That's not really the pits when it happens seldom or in emergency or as a special treat. It's when the kids are habitually given that quick fix of empty calories and sneaky snacks, which, if not all bad for them, at least aren't doing any good in the way of nourishment.

The really sad part of the scenario is that those parents (and grandparents, relatives, and neighbors) are setting the kids up for a lifetime addiction. The "present" for these small fry may not be dope or tobacco or alcohol. But over the long haul a habit is formed and that sugar-coated or fat-filled slop ranks high in the dietary preferences of the child, choices that can eventually shorten his or her life.

As a matter of fact, sometimes we don't have to wait for middle or old age for the outcome. In the last few decades doctors and pediatricians (medical specialists for children) have been able to trace certain ailments appearing in children at least partly to bad food habits that started early on.

They use some heavy words to describe those conditions, such as *hyperkinesia, hyperactivity,* and *hypertonic syn-*

drome. The problems caused by these abnormal conditions cause a continual state of upset for the child and the whole family. Symptoms include excessive physical movement and activity, orneriness, problems in learning, short attention span, and difficulty getting along with other children as well as adults.

Although the theory may call for further study, prominent doctors and researchers are currently concerned with the evidence that what a child eats can make him or her dull or alert, bright or stupid, backward or advanced, obedient or unmanageable. That is not to say that food is the only hero or villain of the piece, but food habits can help, or harm.

Contractors and architects from time to time have been criticized for allowing the use of weak or faulty materials in the construction of buildings and bridges, for example. How many parents are indicted for using sleazy building materials like harmful or junk foods in feeding their kids? Yet the result is very much the same. The "construction" has a short life and iffy service, bridge or child.

It is seldom only lack of information or intelligence on the part of parents who neglect to notice what kids eat or don't eat. Especially when the children are little, few parents neglect doctor visits. But those same parents often find it easier to give in when it comes to the baby's or toddler's screams for inferior or harmful foods. Overseeing the child's intake of the proper foods day after day takes time and effort. We don't let the baby in our charge put his or her hand into a flame or an electrical outlet if we can help it; why do we invariably let the youngster con us into offering sugar crispies instead of a wholesome breakfast?

In this day of sky-high prices, it's actually cheaper for parents to stock the pantry or the refrigerator with items to help instill healthful eating and drinking habits in the family's small ones. Prices of the good and the bad are similar. A few sound substitutions that can be made without bruising the budget include fruit juices instead of soft drinks, raisins for potato chips, and raw fruits and vegetables for candy bars.

The younger that good eating habits are formed, the better: better for the baby, the toddler, the adolescent, the young adult and his or her life span. With wrong or inadequate nutrition, the heart problems, the ugly patches of arteriosclerosis clogging the arteries and threatening their early hardening, can start very, very young.

Fair, Fat, and Fourteen
(or Sixteen, or Eighteen)

If we haven't done it so far, maybe we can get your attention with these three funky "F's." Reliable sources (your age group) tell us that the "fat sixteens" and the "fat eighteens" are as bad as the "fat fourteens." And many child psychologists and psychiatrists now are certain that many adult personality and emotional disorders can be traced directly to the fat fours, the fat sixes, and the fats of all elementary as well as high-school years.

Looking back on our own adolescence, it was among goals in those days to have a slim, well-proportioned body and super-clear skin. Those were, for sure, more important than good grades and high marks on the report card. What clown would expect to win a popular date on his or her scores in math and English? No way.

With a lot of us, proper nutrition got its best shot shortly after we were born. Time was when a young mother would boast of the fact that her infant had weighed nine or even ten pounds at delivery; it was proof positive that she "took care of herself and ate well" during her pregnancy.

Medical advances showed, however, that an overweight mother and an overweight newborn were not all that smooth. Fat mothers more often than not overate on nonnourishing foods. Fat babies often had a tough time entering the world because their size gave problems to the doctor or midwife delivering them. Many obstetricians know today that a delivery weight of six and one-half to seven and one-half pounds is better for the mother and can actually give the baby a better, healthier start in life.

But even today, with all our new medical knowledge, isn't it a status symbol for parents to show off "a fat, healthy baby"? Not really. The myth persists that a fat baby is always healthy. The danger is that the tiny tub of lard is being trained in some very bad eating habits that will last through old age—if the overweight baby ever reaches it.

According to the experts, one of the saddest untruths voiced by parents in response to criticism is: "It's only baby fat; he (she) will outgrow it!" The fact is that fat babies have the best chance of becoming fat toddlers, fat teenagers, and then fat adults. That scenario usually can be reversed only with the help of proper diet combined with proper exercise.

Simply put, the fat little kid is carrying around more fat than he or she should—not necessarily more pounds, because children differ a lot in body build. Parents who suspect that their youngster might be overweight, then, should make an appointment with the pediatrician, not just consult the insurance company's height-and-weight chart. The doctor will know what to prescribe in the way of diet and eating habits, and the parents of such a child need that professional help and advice. Between the ages of about seven and fifteen "baby fat" is expected to melt away as the child grows in height. It *can* happen. However, the child who is downright overweight before the age of seven, and certainly after fifteen or sixteen, can be in big trouble in the future unless helped back to normal or near-normal weight.

We can't nag too often that gross overweight means a severe health hazard at any age. It puts a real strain on the heart and blood vessels, which worsens as the fat remains or builds up. Nor have the organs of the rest of the body been programmed to take care of the burden. Overweight can also be a factor in bringing on or worsening diabetes, a special scourge of the teens.

In a nation and a generation that seem to demand "think

thin," even skinny, things can get hairy in the adolescent and early adult years. We all want to be accepted, to have our company sought out among our peers. The overweight, particularly the obese, in the teen years often can't handle it when they don't make the scene among classmates and friends. Controlled scientific studies of the problem have been made among young people in summer camps and junior and senior high school students. The overweight girls seemed to have the worst hang-ups: They tended to isolate themselves from their peers; they withdrew into family life, but found that a drag; they were less outgoing and social; they were obsessed with the thought of food and what it might be doing to their physical shape and popularity. Rather than being interested in learning about nutrition, they thought of just plain eating. That brought a reaction that was a kind of guilt trip, a kind of wicked, sinful preoccupation.

For the most part, the slim girls of the same age groups were more relaxed, extraverted, and sociable and looked on food and eating more as an all-right, normal, and involuntary occupation.

The boys were a little less obviously disturbed, but the chubbies of both sexes were unhappy and upset, lacked self-esteem, and were resentful of themselves and the world around them for their being fat. Their lot, they felt in varying degrees, was the loneliness of unpopularity, being a figure of fun and even dislike and disgust, an outcast.

The Dreary Drama of the Diet Pill

You don't have to visit a famine-suffering, underdeveloped Third World nation to see dwarfism caused by malnutrition. Pediatricians and other medical specialists have seen too many American children who never would reach their full height and weight because they were short-changed on nutrition at a critical time.

Young girls in the early period of menstruation need all the iron they can get to replace that lost monthly through menstrual flow. When they "diet" by swearing off whole-grain or enriched breads and iron-laden vegetables, they are really asking for anemia, the starvation of red blood cells, leaving them inadequate in quality and quantity to fight disease.

Recently some scientists have stressed the belief that avoidance of physical activity and all kinds of exercise can be a bigger villain than the calories totted up in the foods young people eat. The setup is clear. Fat kids are seldom if ever chosen for the softball or volley ball team. If they go out for swimming, they're gross and self-conscious in a swim suit. Some really heavy kids complain that just walking hurts. The result? The fatties stay in, stay covered, stay near the food, stay in front of the tube, which offers no criticism about form or figure (except in the commercials with "diet aids" and slim models). All this neatly wards off the danger of peer rejection from the outside.

Just a few words on "diet pills," "reducing candies," "appetite suppressants," call 'em what you will. Actually most are forms of artificial uppers, which alter and eventually damage the body's chemical balance.

Unfortunately, those dumb pills can be sold over the counter, without a prescription. Often there's no minimum age for purchasers, and even if there were, it would be tough these days for a salesman or pharmacist to judge who's over and who's under the magic eighteen years of age. That means that some kids in their early teens can find it a piece of cake to walk off with the pills if they can come up with the bread to waste.

Down the road, if the pills alter or harm the body chemistry they can be very dangerous to life and health. In the short run, they can cause painful and unpleasant side effects: insomnia, excessively dry mouth, stepped-up heartbeat, irritability. Overdoing them can have bizarre results in altering or ruining the body's natural metabolism, probably for life.

Such pills can also be addictive. Some studies have found

that when users stop taking the drugs—and they are just that—they suffer a severe let-down feeling and actual withdrawal symptoms.

That's the worst part, for your present and future health. But even if the pills weren't harmful to your body, they are to your budget. And even if they were free, they just don't work as far as melting off pounds is concerned.

Believe it or not, things were once worse. Diet pills have been around for a long time. There have always been fat people who wanted the miracle of slimness achieved suddenly with some magic pill or potion.

Until 1979 the nation was deluged with the promotion of what pharmacists call "sympathomimetic amines." In rough translation, those are drugs that stimulate the central nervous system; they turn down the appetite through action on the centers of the brain involved.

Then the Congress passed the Drug Abuse Prevention and Control Act, which reclassified many drugs. It had the effect of suppressing some of them both in manufacture and circulation. Amphetamines (sound familiar?), stimulants in the form of drugs, combined with tranquilizers and sedatives had been banned in 1973.

But the smart guys got around the rules and laws with substitute preparations. The "new" ones have a lot in common with the originals. Now as then, they don't live up to the promise they make, and they can bring on those nasty side effects. And many of you young adults, longing for the form divine and glamorous dates from an overnight pill miracle, are or will be among their most reliable customers.

Medical consultants agree: The best course for the high-schooler and for everyone, and what is easiest on health and the wallet, is cutting down on fattening and nonnourishing foods, eating well-balanced and nourishing meals, and getting plenty of sensible exercise. Dull, but in most cases it really works.

Pimples Are the Pits

O.K., by now you should know a little about general nourishment, metabolism, and how a stupid crash diet or habit-forming reducing pills can ruin your prospects—or shorten your life.

Well, there's this great guy or gal in English Comp. who makes it tough for you to concentrate on the agreement of subject and verb. Most of your daydreams involve a spectacular conquest of your secret idol.

But in real life you have little or no hope for that happy ending. Shattering your romantic dream is the cold, cruel fact that on your adoring face there are pimples—and blackheads and whiteheads. Who would find groovy and attractive a mug that looks like a relief map of Ireland, you ask?

First of all, knock off feeling sorry for yourself as a far-out freak. You're not at all "different." If that's your plight, you've got lots of company. Doctors figure that 86 percent of American adolescents and young people suffer from the skin ailment called acne by the time they reach seventeen years of age.

But teens and young adults don't make up the whole picture. Almost half of those who see a doctor or dermatologist about acne are past twenty years of age, and a third of American women between twenty and fifty suffer from some form of acne.

You're right in what you're probably thinking. The fact that the greater part of the population has or has had the misery of acne—skin eruptions known through generations as "hickies" —doesn't help *your problem.*

Physiology and adolescent development being the facts of life that they are, we have little doubt that in ancient civilizations nature struck young victims with acne. An Egyptian medical textbook, believed to be about 3,000 years old, has a whole section on skin and scalp disorders; age or age groups are not mentioned, but it's a cinch that some of the ailments discussed centered about what we know today as "adolescent acne."

That's a flaky word, acne; where did we latch on to it? Actually, it is adapted from the Greek word *akne* meaning "eruption on the face." Many ailments and diseases have names adapted from early Greek or Latin words.

Chances are that what really sends you up the wall is the fact that the uglies set up housekeeping mainly on your face, just the part you can't hide with sexy jeans or T-shirts.

There's a reason for that. It has to do with how you're made and how you grow and develop into young adulthood. Let's talk a little about the construction of the skin, the whole skin, and nothing but the skin. It might help you understand how it all happens.

First of all, we have said that the skin is the largest organ of the body, protecting as well as covering the whole frame. It's just as complex as the other vital organs of the body, but for our purposes let's consider it as made up of two main layers: the bottom layer, known as the *dermis*, and the top layer, covering the surface, called the *epidermis*. Once more, the Greeks had a word, or words, for it: *Derm* in Greek means "skin," and *epi* means "over."

The epidermis is actually the thin but sturdy outermost covering of the body, which acts as an overall protection for more fragile parts against any enemy from the outside world: infection, wound, severe heat, or severe cold.

The dermis, about five times as thick as the outer layer, has a number of main structures, including capillaries (little blood vessels surrounding each sweat gland); nerve endings (the skin's alert signals to sudden change, as in temperature and pressure); hair follicles (pockets holding growing hairs); fat deposits (cushions against bumps and frigid cold); oil glands (whose oil keeps the skin and hair soft), and sweat glands, which throw off waste water in the form of perspiration.

The two types of glands, sweat and oil, have different ways of doing their job. Sweat glands, as noted, throw off liquid wastes onto the surface of the skin; they remove the discards from the skin capillaries and shoot them into the channels of the glands, which jet them onto the skin through the pores at the ends of the channels. Their openings, very near the surface, are too tiny to be seen with the naked eye.

Oil glands, or *sebaceous glands*, do their own thing. Their assignment is to keep the skin soft and supple by lubricating it. They deliver their oil into *follicles*, or "pores." The follicles, shaped like tiny tubes, carry the oil from the sebaceous glands to the surface of the skin.

There are millions of oil glands and sweat glands all over the skin of the body. But the oil glands and pores are more concentrated in the skin of the face, back, and chest. On the face, certain sections of skin contain as many as 2,000 oil glands to a square inch. (The palms of the hands and the soles of the feet have no oil glands; that's probably why they look soggy and wrinkled as a prune after soaking in water for a while.)

Let's look now at how dead cells are discarded to make room for new ones. Maybe you've seen your mother or a dressmaker fold back the end of a piece of fabric to form a lining. It's like that with the walls of the follicles: the walls are really the continued extension of the epidermis; the epidermis turns in and down to line the follicles.

Old cells rising to the surface of the skin through the follicles flatten out as they die. The dead cells are continually sloughed off, and their places are taken by fresh cells coming up from the lower to the top area of the epidermis. In brief, the lining of the follicles produces new cells, which die, drop into the follicle, and then are pushed out to the surface of the skin, where they flake off. (The flaking-off stuff is called *keratin*; you can sometimes see it on dark clothes. Keratin is not dandruff, although it resembles it; dandruff is a different story.)

As long as things flow along smoothly like this, all is well. When the system breaks down or gets tangled somehow, acne can happen.

For instance, it's a bad scene when the cells that line the follicle stay stuck together, as opposed to flowing outward toward the surface of the skin. The cells don't separate but start to build up along the follicle wall, and the wall begins to thicken and bulge.

This failure of free-flow can mean plugged up or clogged follicles caused by dead cells and oil.

What happens? Acne. And that means pimples, blackheads, whiteheads, cysts, blotches, or small red bumps. Many doctors and dermatologists call this kind of acne "a disease of plugged follicles." Whatever it's called, to you it's just plain ugly.

Until not too long ago, there didn't seem to be much we could do about it. Grin and bear it (wait until you "grow out" of it) seemed to be the usual dreary advice, but it is very hard to grin and far from easy trying to "bear" it.

But recently we've found out a little more about how it starts and progresses. Some dermatologists point out that, like so many troubles in life, the initial "plug" starts out tiny. At first we can scarcely see any of the plugs, partly because we're not looking for them. They are, in effect, "baby pimples." Right now, it's believed that if we can keep those little plugs from growing and developing, we can get a jump on a serious acne condition.

The "treatment" seems simple and relatively cheap. You wash your face *gently* (don't rub and scrub) with a pure mild soap or a good cleanser that doesn't contain oil. Then in some cases you apply a drying/peeling agent or medication to the skin. You can wash your face as often as you think necessary, but don't forget to reapply the medication, which really does all the work.

The drying/peeling medication can break apart the dead cells that are sticking together in the pores; it discourages the forming of such plugs and breaks up some that have already gotten a start.

There are other treatments that for our purpose we need not go into: antibiotics, cortisone, ultraviolet light, peeling treatments, X ray, injections, and more. For any of those, don't try to go it alone without professional guidance. If you or your family are considering any of them, see your family doctor and let him or her help make the decision. Maybe you'll be advised to see a dermatologist, maybe the doctor will have some answers for your particular case if it's not serious. The point is, in severe cases especially, don't try to treat yourself. You may do much damage.

Speaking of damage, for pete's sake, try to keep your hands away from your face. Squeezing pimples and blackheads and whiteheads can only harm, not help, your problem. It can cause long-standing or permanent scars, or your fingers can spread the infection and break delicate capillaries near the surface of the skin. Fingers, incidentally, should be clean at all times, particularly in the case of acne.

Now for the acne scene itself, past and present.

Until a generation or so ago, parents and elders—even the doctor—were sure as shootin' that diet was Hit Man Number One that brought on and worsened acne, especially certain foods favored by teens and young people.

High on the list of no-no's have been chocolate, fatty and fried foods, potato chips, cola drinks, all kinds of "sweets," and all kinds of nuts.

You can understand the suspicion, because most of those items had been neatly inserted into the junk food slot. Would you believe that also on the enemy list, at some time or other, were dairy products, carrots, citrus fruits, tomatoes and tomato products, shellfish, even spinach, cabbage, lettuce, and artichokes?

Since the early bad-guys list, the last-named have been cleared of their bad reputation in the acne argument because it was found that they contain useful vitamins and minerals.

At present, many dermatologists are saying flatly that no one item, or combination of items, can be responsible for acne. They say, further, that since adolescence and young adulthood is a critical period of growth and development, there's no reason to combat acne with the single weapon of depriving the sufferer or potential sufferer of certain dietary items. He or she needs all the food building-blocks to be had.

C H A P T E R • V

The Jury on Junk

You know that your body needs, daily, certain chemical nutrients. Nutrition experts have put them all into six basic types: carbohydrates, proteins, fats, vitamins, minerals, and water. (Most people don't think of water as "nutritious," but it is vital to metabolism. Water is the liquid in which all the chemical reactions of the living material in the cell take place. Every one of the cells contains water; it carries nutrients to all of the cells; it carries wastes away; it helps keep the body at the proper temperature.)

The six types of nutrients are critical not only to your role as top high school athlete but also to all your daily ho-hum schedules and chores. Would you believe those nutrients also play a role in getting you through that lousy math quiz?

Not turned on? O.K., let's talk about the ingredients that go into typical junk and fast foods. As far as nourishment goes, whether you receive an allowance or have a job to help pick up the tab, someone's hard-earned money is really going down the tube for that gulped hamburger or hot dog.

Consider the all-American hot dog. (We're not calling all brands on the carpet, particularly not some kosher or "chicken" franks.) Outside of the paper-thin hamburger, slapped together with "fillers" without which it would be inedible, the first place on your meat-snack list is the hot dog. What "binders" and "extenders" are used in the frank? Items like starch, soy flour, and dried milk—not harmful, but certainly substituting empty calories for the protein (an essential food component) you should be getting with any meat intake.

Forget the soggy, nonnourishing white bun and the inferior mustard or relish. Let's concentrate on the content of the frankfurter.

The "meat" in hot dogs is often just the discard trimmed from ham and chops. If any "red meat" sneaks in, it is usually tiny bits clinging to the big hunks of fat. If any protein is present, it is in the slight amount of dried milk or soy flour.

The discard-ingredients are crushed and beaten together and then kneaded with the fat, water, and additives, creating a mudlike dough. The mush is stuffed into a sausage-shaped casing or skin coated with a bright red artificial coloring. Oxidizing chemicals used for curing (processing) meat speed up the cooking and intensify the red color.

Manufacturers of some hot dog brands use parts of muscle meat and a great deal of animal fat; some factories use pork stomachs, jowls, salivary glands, lymph nodes, and cheek fats. It's not downright illegal to use the trash. And it's hard, if not impossible, to list the ingredients on the individual frank that you are handed at the lunch counter or in the school cafeteria.

How much protein do you suppose that "meat product" gives you? Nutritionists say, at the rate we've spelled out, that many brands of hot dog measure up something like this: 56 percent water, 28 percent fat, 12 percent protein, and 4 percent "other."

Never mind the short-changing on the protein. How would you feel about a hash dish your mom cooked up for dinner consisting of a tiny bit of ham or corned beef, a lot of water, much fat or suet that she usually throws out—and snips and snails and puppy dogs' tails? Not too cool!

Don't take our word for it. Study the weird tales about "what's in a hot dog" as reported by such reputable journals as *Consumer Reports*, or the testimony of U.S. Department of Agriculture officials before congressional hearings. That's where we got our evidence.

Back to the heaven we call hamburger. Misleading name, to begin with: The burger doesn't get it from the "ham" it doesn't contain. Back in the Stone Age to you (about the turn of the century), "hamburg" was chopped beef from top- or bottom-round steak. Simply translated, that meant good and nutritionally sound beef. Think of today's version. All it takes is a little common sense. At today's prices of good, protein-filled beef, how much of that do you suppose the fast-food chain puts into its burgers? Right. As little as it can get away with and with as much nothingness "filler" as it can manage short of arrest for fraud and downright toxicity. Yet tight as the family finances may be, the American young adult, perhaps more than any other segment of society, continues to build both the popularity and the fortunes of the fast-food hamburger kings.

There's no need to consult the charts to measure nourishment in either the hot dog or the hamburger. What you're getting for your money are mainly water and fat and filler. In terms of nutrients, just about zilch.

The Cola Connection

How often do you see the young person of high-school age portrayed by media ads without a soft drink in his or her hand? Watch your TV commercials.

Soft drinks aren't all that soft. The hard fact is that the three big C's—coffee, cocoa, and cola—have something harsh in common. Their main ingredient is a not-so-little number known as *caffeine*, a hype to your nervous system that can give you an artificial up; it is also suspected of causing certain birth defects in children of mothers who have overindulged during pregnancy.

The story goes that the discovery of caffeine as a sleep preventer dates back to an ancient Arabian monastery. Some shepherds herding goats saw their charges eating coffee beans and then later watched those same goats run around energetically all night long. The shepherds told their tale to the head of the monastery, and it gave him an idea. Something in the coffee beans kept the goats up all night, he figured, and he made a drink from the beans to keep him awake for the long night hours when he wanted to be alert for his prayers.

Caffeine, unless prescribed by the doctor for medicinal purposes, is not good for either man or beast. A stimulant drug, it is found in large quantities in tea leaves, coffee beans, and kola nuts. In addition, the kola bean, for example, is so bitter that soft drinks in which it is used must contain lots of sugar to be drinkable.

But caffeine has enjoyed a pretty good career as an "additive." Today it is used as a so-called additive in several soft drinks close to the young adult heart.

Although the kola bean in its native state contains a great deal of caffeine, much of it is processed out to make a saleable softie. So the processor or manufacturer seems to feel dutybound to put it back in order to give the young drinker spark, hype, whatever. Some colas must contain caffeine because of the very nature of the beast; there's no law that says it must be mentioned in the list of ingredients. Some other carbonated soft drinks contain caffeine, but that content has to be included on the label.

Let's see how the caffeine content in various drinks and pills stacks up, according to a recent chart of the U.S. Food and Drug Administration. It tells us that one average-size cup of coffee contains about 90 milligrams of caffeine. (A milligram is 0.001 of a gram, or 0.015 grains.) Uppers like "wakeup" pills can contain about 110 milligrams of caffeine. Cola drinks are not too far behind, containing 40 to 72 milligrams to the 12-ounce bottle or can.

Caffeine hypes up children and teens more than it does adults, because the adults have more resistance and less sensitivity. Thus it takes a greater and quicker toll in making the youngster abnormally nervous and hyperactive.

The average American (including many young adults) is

hooked on both coffee and other caffeine-laden drinks. Some nutritionists believe that the addiction is the main reason why the sales of tranquilizers and downers continue to soar annually.

The score isn't final on all studies and researches on caffeine, but we do know that it speeds up production of stomach acid and is among suspected villains in causing peptic ulcer, which is caused by an increased jetting of digestive juices into the stomach.

What we do know for sure is that persons who drink large quantities of coffee daily may come down with a real, low-grade illness popularly known as "caffeinism," causing insomnia, rise in temperature, and constant irritability. These symptoms are reduced or stop altogether when the intake of coffee decreases or stops.

So we suggest that you think over these facts the next time you have an urge for a second mug of coffee or another cola. You can't beat water: It's good for you, it contains no calories, and best of all, it really quenches that thirst.

The Gyp of the Chip

With all the foodstuffs you buy, junk or otherwise, we can't warn too often: Read the labels!

You probably know that, by law, ingredients are listed by quantity on labels. What the item contains most of is listed first, and so on down the line. A glance at the label of the average bag of potato chips reads: potato, vegetable oil, partially hydrogenized soybean oil, salt. That adds up to very little, if any, in nutrients.

Like caffeine, the potato chip has had its movers and shakers. In the late nineteenth century an American Indian named George Crum (no kidding), working in the kitchen of a hotel in Saratoga Springs, New York, experimented with deep-frying some raw potatoes sliced paper-thin. He began to serve the new product, and it caught on as "potato chips."

Things were relatively harmless while the hotel guest could, for example, order potato chips for a snack in the dining room. Despite the deep fat in which they were fried, the customer was getting a little phosphorus (mineral), iron, and vitamins. But by the early twentieth century, manufacturers of potato chips saw the promise of big business and big profits. They foresaw, correctly, that much of the potential was in the child and high-school-age markets.

However, the chips were on the frail side, easily broken, and perhaps worst of all for the maker, had a "short shelf life." They turned rancid and stale or spoiled quickly. Something had to be done to correct these negatives.

Problem followed problem for fast-fooders who wanted to turn a fast buck. Inflation, soaring since the early 1970's, created high prices for all foods, which threatened to shrink sales on such snacks as chips, and costs of all ingredients continued to rise.

Then a light appeared at the end of the processing tunnel. Dehydrated (water-removed) potatoes could be used as a restructured chip, and the dehydrates, of course, could be of a much cheaper grade of potato. Besides, the "restructureds" were beginning to sell well as a novelty. The old school of potato-chip making and the "restructionists" did battle with promotion to increase sales. Even the Food and Drug Administration got into the fray, but not into the full-scale war, and the status remained quo.

The new and modern (not nutritionally improved) chips are probably here to stay in this plastic age. With their innocence of nutrition they are, in effect, more costly and less flavorful than conceived by George Crum. As it turned out, despite Crum's American heritage, his invention became un-American nutritionally in a make-believe world of promotion and distribution. In some instances the name potato chip has been dropped altogether from the product: witness Ruffles, Pringles, you name it.

A Look At Fast-Food Nutrients*

The following tables list nutritive values of foods available at some fast-food restaurant chains. The data were based on nutritional analyses made in recent years by the chains themselves and printed in the March-April 1981 issue of *Dietetic Currents*. For simplication, the data were converted by *FDA Consumer* into percentages of the U.S. Recommended Daily Allowances (U.S. RDAs). FDA requires U.S. RDA information on nutrition labels of many foods. The specific chains are not identified in the tables because the material does not cover the entire fast-food industry. However, the information is intended to give the reader an idea of the nutritive values of fast foods.

HAMBURGERS

	Chain A	Chain B	Chain C
Serving Size (g)	91	102	97
Calories	244	255	263
Protein (g)	11	12	13
Carbohydrates (g)	29	30	29
Fat (g)	9	10	11
Cholesterol (mg)	27	25	26
Sodium (mg)	N/A	520	566

Percent of U.S. RDA (for adults and children over 4 years):

Protein	17%	19%	20%
Vitamin A	2%	-	-
Vitamin C	2%	3%	-
Thiamine	11%	17%	18%
Riboflavin	9%	11%	11%
Niacin	14%	20%	28%
Calcium	5%	5%	8%
Iron	11%	13%	13%

MILKSHAKES

	Chain A	Chain B	Chain C
Serving Size (g)	336	291	322
Calories	403	383	325
Protein (g)	10	10	11
Carbohydrates (g)	72	66	55
Fat (g)	9	9	7
Cholesterol (mg)	36	30	26
Sodium (mg)	N/A	300	270

Percent of U.S. RDA (for adults and children over 4 years):

Protein	15%	15%	17%
Vitamin A	6%	7%	N/A
Vitamin C	-	-	5%
Thiamine	11%	8%	11%
Riboflavin	45%	26%	38%
Niacin	2%	3%	3%
Calcium	45%	32%	35%
Iron	6%	4%	4%

FRENCH FRIES

	Chain A	Chain B	Chain C
Serving Size (g)	68	68	71
Calories	250	220	200
Protein (g)	2	3	2
Carbohydrates (g)	20	26	25
Fat (g)	19	12	10
Cholesterol (mg)	0	9	N/A
Sodium (mg)	N/A	109	N/A

*SOURCE: Reprinted from the May 1983 *FDA Consumer*. HHS Publication No. (FDA) 77-2083. U.S. Department of Health and Human Services.

THE QUICK FIX OF CONVENIENCE FOODS

A new question comes up a great deal, mostly in adult conversations but sometimes in school if you have a nutrition course. The question goes something like this: Did our grandparents and great-grandparents eat better and more nutritionally than we do today?

On the one hand, so the argument goes, the soil in which grandma's fruits and vegetables were grown contained more minerals and other nutrients than the worn-out soil of today. Moreover, people of previous generations picked and ate much of that produce "fresh," as opposed to buying it maybe a week or more later after cross-country trucks have transported it to the supermarket.

On the other hand, it's true that we have infinitely more knowledge about food and nutrition than we did decades ago. But some nutritionists say that this improved knowledge has worked out to little or no benefit to the consumer. They argue that whatever gains were to be had were deposited in the bank accounts of food processors, food transporters, and manufacturers of food substitutes.

Starting with Square One as we see it, our main quarrel is with the food processors who put substitutes, additives, coloring, and "stretchers" into the packaged foods our parents buy. A lot of it has to do with "preservatives," nonnourishing substances that add days and weeks and months to an item's "shelf life."

Frozen, processed, and dehydrated foods have become a way of life, but the additives, the colorings, and the stretchers are not cheap. As a matter of fact, considering the lack of food value that they cover up, they turn out to be mighty expensive.

Let's take one popular item. Among the favorite fall-backs for the "busy" parent is "instant soup." By the time it gets into your soup bowl it's mostly water that you provide courtesy of the tap in the kitchen sink. Nutrition researchers point out

what your mom is getting and giving when she serves a helping of the average brand of "instant soup"; corn starch (used
in the manufacture of paste), hydrogenated (added hydrogen)
vegetable oil, lactose (lactic acid), salt, natural flavors, freeze-
dried chicken meat, chicken fat, dehydrated onion, sugar. The
list goes on and on with very little or nothing that could be
actually classified as "food," let alone nourishment.

The sad fact is that, since the package is *labeled* with the
"ingredients," the law has been obeyed. In the listing of the
ingredients, the one present in the largest quantity is listed
first; the second largest quantity second, and so on. When
colorings or additives are used they are usually listed (but not
by quantity). In explaining their presence, coy phrases are
used like "Added to retain texture," or "Added to retard
spoilage." Roughly translated, that means that the substance
is used to postpone the time when the product goes bad and is
completely unusable.

This is all under governmental regulation, which does not
really seem to be on the consumer's side, when you consider
it.

In the long run, despite the fact that it might require less
time and energy for the one preparing meals, "convenience
food" usually translates into an advantage mainly to the processor and his shareholders.

Several writers on nutrition assert that food processors
operate on the premise that they can turn a profit by their
outright fabrication of foods and useless additives. But, they
argue, wholesome nourishment through *real* foods could well
bring in profits along with an advantage for the consumer.

The opinion is increasingly widespread among profession-
als that the two bureaucratic giants on which we consumers
depend for nutrition information—the Food and Drug
Administration and the Department of Agriculture—have
done, and continue to do, less than a great job for us. The two
bureaus are accused by some nutritionists of making little
effort to prevent adulteration and use of inferior ingredients
in some of our foods.

Chances are that as a young adult, still living at home, you have little say in what comes from the supermarket and stocks the larder. But you do about the treats and snacks you buy for yourself. Maybe you've never looked at the ingredients listed on your candy bars, your potato chips, your soda bottles or cans. Even though they don't give you the truth, the whole truth, and nothing but, read the ingredients on labels. It's high time you started the habit.

Food Fads, Food Foolishness

What is a "fad diet"? A diet prescribed and supervised by a physician makes some sense. The doctor can tailor a diet to our individual needs in the way of nourishing foods and foods to avoid. In fact, the traditional daily diet includes all or most of the nutrients to meet the body's basic needs.

On the other hand, the fad diet is one that goes along with the purple prose on the dust jackets of countless books these days: the quick-fix diet that "guarantees" that in a few weeks (sometimes days!) it will give you a slim waist, disappearing thighs, and chest measurements that will be the envy of a fashion model.

Food fads, as such, have been around for a long time. Looking at the picture historically, billions of people of all cultures over the centuries and millennia have been prey to the slick, silver-tongued pusher interested only in the fast buck.

The ancient Egyptians may have been among the earliest food faddists. They doled out generous supplies of garlic daily (their recipe for physical strength) to feed slaves and other workers building the pyramids. About 3600 B.C., "nutritional" applications of sliced lettuce were made to the scalp to encourage hair growth on young men threatened with baldness.

From time to time, one- or two-food diets have been advanced with two prime goals: fantastic benefits of super health and long life and the "immediate benefit" of fast weight loss.

In the 1940's and 1950's those two great results were promised for grapefruit and avocado. (Comparatively, there's little nourishment in either fruit, but a great deal of water.) At the same time, the diets advised by some health and beauty magazines (then as now devoured by collegians) were heavy on expensive cuts of lean meat and hard-to-get, out-of-season vegetables.

The fad diets of the 1980's to provide "nourishment" and to avoid such nasties as colds and calories call for extra amounts of certain commercially produced vitamins and delicious "cocktails" such as vinegar and honey combinations to keep the internal plumbing clean and strong. There's nothing terribly wrong with honey; it's an energy source, but fattening. However, large amounts of vinegar in beverages can help dry up the very "pipes" (veins and arteries) we're warned to help keep healthy and vigorous.

Right now, the big danger is popular diets that promise the sun, the moon, and the stars but deliver mostly bread to the wallets of the guys who dream them up. Diet books crowd the shelves of bookstores, and the publisher in most cases gets the lion's share of the take.

Dr. Mark Hegsted, a well-known nutritionist, in a recent article in *Health* magazine, made a careful analysis of the more popular diets. He stressed that the one thing we know for sure about diets and overweight is that "to lose body fat you must see to it that your total caloric intake is less than the amount of energy you expend."

The American passion for "one great gimmick" to make the problem easy is a great ally of gullibility, according to Dr. Hegsted. He adds:

"But losing weight and maintaining proper weight are obviously *not* easy in our society. If they were, the problem long since would have been solved and the market for new diets would disappear along with obesity. In fact, we can be sure that when there are many solutions offered for the same problem, none of them is very satisfactory."

Dr. Hegsted's analysis, briefly stated, appears in the accompanying chart, "The Diets at a Glance." As can be seen, none of them is completely satisfactory for any young adult, particularly in the nourishment department.

In this do-it-yourself-book age, it's a little like shooting fish in a barrel to steer buyers of diet books to the cashier. No doubt the fish most targeted are thirtyish and middle-aged women, but too many are teens and young adults of both sexes.

The Diets at a Glance*

DIET	WHAT PRIN- CIPLE IS IN- VOLVED?	IS THE DIET SAFE?	IS THE DIET EASY TO STICK TO?	ARE THE FOODS INEX- PENSIVE, EASY TO FIND, ETC.?	CAN THE WHOLE FAMILY EAT THIS DIET?	WILL IT GIVE YOU GOOD LONG- TERM EATING HABITS?
The Never- Say-Diet Diet	Reduced calories, limited choice, more exer- cise	Yes	Yes	Yes	Foods yes, amounts no	Yes
The Beverly Hills Diet	Fruit only	No	No	Expensive and at times hard to obtain	No	No
The University Diet	Two low- calorie meals, one low-calorie supple- ment drink per day	Yes	No	Yes	No	Probably not
The Cambridge Diet	330 calo- ries per day	No	No	Yes	No	No
The Atkins Diet	High-fat, low-carbo- hydrate intake; ketosis	Not nutri- tionally balanced; too much fat	Not very easy	Easily available, possibly costly	No	No

The Diets at a Glance*

DIET	WHAT PRINCIPLE IS INVOLVED?	IS THE DIET SAFE?	IS THE DIET EASY TO STICK TO?	ARE THE FOODS INEXPENSIVE, EASY TO FIND, ETC.?	CAN THE WHOLE FAMILY EAT THIS DIET?	WILL IT GIVE YOU GOOD LONG-TERM EATING HABITS?
The Stillman Diet	High protein intake	Not nutritionally balanced	Not very easy	Demands careful shopping, a lot of meat purchases	No	No
The Scarsdale Diet	Reduced calories, limited choice	Yes	Not in the long run	Easy to find, easy to prepare, but costly	Foods yes, amounts no	Maybe
The Pritkin Diet	Radically reduced intake of calories, fats, protein, sugar, salt	Yes	Not very easy	Inexpensive and easy to find but calls for whole new approach to shopping, cooking	Maybe	Yes

*From *Health* Magazine, January 1983.

Competition for success on all fronts among the young adult age groups is at an all-time high. Actually, the quest for the starved look far outweighs that of parent-pleasing school grades or popularity at sports.

Upping the ante for shots at this age group is that many young adults develop a positive passion for physical fitness. What starts off as a national fitness campaign may reverse for the young adult into a fad diet that is eventually self-defeating and even self-destructive.

Chub Gregson had just marked his eighteenth birthday when his mail brought a notification that his application had been accepted to one of the top Ivy League colleges. What's more, a partial academic scholarship he was sure of getting could mean that his dad's dream of a financial career for Chub would turn into reality.

His son had other ambitions. Those turned more to catching the eye of a scout representing a good team with the National Football League—because the school granting degrees in business administration also had a crack football team.

Chub's dream at that point was to be there when the college team's football tryouts began. One big cloud. As you might guess from his nickname, Chub had a weight problem, and as things stood, he was afraid he had about as much chance as a snowball in August of being considered for frosh football.

What to do? Not to worry. Chub's pal, Bucky Miller, already enrolled in a local college, had always been the idea man in the high school crowd. A little embarrassed, Chub talked the problem over with Bucky, who asked his friend to give him a little time. For the first time in memory, Bucky showed an interest in his mother's magazines. It didn't take him long to spot an article with the catchy title "Be Slim, Be Sexy." It detailed a sure-fire diet that promised a loss of nineteen pounds in fifteen days. All Chub had to do, Bucky told him, was to follow an easy eating pattern:

Breakfast: a small glass of orange juice and a cup of black coffee. Lunch: dry toast and an apple. Dinner: another cup of black coffee and a small dish of canned fruit. Snacks could include two diet soft drinks spaced out through the day. (Breakfast and lunch would be easy, Bucky offered, with the family on staggered hours; at dinner time, a no-show or a "not hungry right now," if questioned.)

Four hungry lonely weeks followed for Chub before he left for college. The loneliness was self-chosen. His dietary program got flak from the family—the future football running-back had been known to his kid sister, Kim, as "Greedy Gus." The usual rap sessions at the corner soda store or the fast-food emporium were out, to avoid temptation.

Chub lost 15 pounds during that month of misery. He also lost his even disposition, his high school friends (except

Bucky, in on the deal), the energy essential for football scrim-
mage, and his until-now famous sense of humor. Greedy Gus
seemed to have had a personality change into Gloomy Gus.
In one short month his body's store of fat cells were gone
and Chub had made himself a likely candidate for malnutrition. A bad scene for any age, his nutrition scam was a catas-
trophe for a still-growing eighteen-year-old. Off in very slow
motion to school, by the time he arrived, Chub had neither
the energy nor interest to report to the football coach at the
time set for tryout.

The story has a delayed happy ending. Nosy kid sister, her
curiosity sharper than her parents', spied doggedly until she
had figured out what Chub had been doing (or not doing) in
the mindless month preparing for football ambitions. With
Chub finally out of the house and college started, Kim alerted
the parents, who had been frankly worried as well as puzzled.
Now somewhat relieved that their son hadn't contracted some
strange form of anorexia nervosa, they nervously waited until
he came home for his winter holiday. Alarmed more at his
listlessness than his wasted body, they sought the advice of a
nutritionist friend. A strategy was planned to expose Chub to
some informal education in sensible nutrition.

It worked. Not only was the starvation diet abandoned, but
Chub also accepted the low-down on how to eat moderately
without the distraction of hunger pains and to get all the
nutrients he needed without looking like a tub of lard. By
spring he had recaptured his natural energy and could
approach the football coach with a fair amount of confidence.

The rest is sports history. Chub (now "Charles" to his professors and "Chuck" to his chums) two years later was responsible for the flocking of pro football recruiters to the college
town to watch him in action.

Chuck is still in his junior year, and it's too early to predict
if one of the pro recruiters might recommend him to a major
league team. At the moment his love for computer courses has

him keeping an eye on his dad's financial hints. Whatever happens, Chuck is in training with proper food and sensible exercise not only for the roar of the gridiron crowds, but for his potential adult life, Wall Street or wherever.

Scenarios of Self-destruction

Wendy Lewis, college sophomore, was bright and attractive through her freshman year, got along with fellow students and professors, seemed destined for the fast-popularity lane of life. Her grades were good, and she enjoyed most classes.

One of her features was a very round face, to parents and teachers a "real baby face," but to her a "gross fat mug."

Toward the end of her freshman year, she made her Number One priority a campaign to melt away the hated fat on that "baby face." Maybe the rest of her wasn't so disgusting, but after all, the face was the first part of her anatomy given the once-over by any new guy.

It started with a few carrot and celery sticks or an occasional half-apple as a substitute for meals, and it went on for about six months.

That spring during intersession, Wendy's parents came for a visit. Wendy went to the airport to meet them, but when she spotted them and called "Mom" and "Dad," they recognized only the familiar voice. The rest of their cherished Wendy seemed to have undergone a radical change. In a word, she now was skinny and gaunt.

It was a brief visit, but the three had a few meals together. The parents were hungry after their long flight, but Wendy picked at her plate and ate just about nothing. She "wasn't hungry" just then, she told her parents. They concluded that she had been hitting the books too hard, and they begged her to let up on studies and night life.

The irony of the situation was that Wendy's concerned dad was a leading pediatrician in their home city. But Dr. Lewis saw mostly infants and toddlers as patients. Neither parent recognized the symptoms of the young-adult ailment anorexia nervosa in Wendy during their brief visit.

Wendy's pursuit of a college degree was interrupted that summer. A sharp young college instructor had been studying nutrition and young eating lapses. Her concern grew as she watched Wendy lose incredible weight; with the dean's permission, she got in touch with Wendy's parents and told them of her suspicions.

The story has a (rare) happy ending. Over her protests that nothing was wrong, Wendy was hospitalized for a few months under professional treatment—psychological as well as dietary. She recovered and lost only half a year from college. Today, the anorexic horror well behind her, Wendy holds a responsible post with a computer firm on the West Coast—and better yet, she eats hearty, well-balanced meals and jogs and bicycles daily.

The Bad News of Bulimia

Another eating disorder is associated with young adults and collegians. Called bulimia, it is not an exact counterpart of anorexia, but it could be called a second stage in the progression of noneating.

In a way, the two disorders seem diametrically opposed: the anorexics avoiding food with a passion, the bulimics wolfing down great quantities of food and immediately getting rid of it. Both groups have a dread of becoming overweight or obese.

The person suffering from bulimia gets the taste and enjoyment of food for a few moments, then takes bizarre steps to make certain no calories do their worst. Generally a girl in her late teens, the bulimic stuffs down foods high in caloric content, then deliberately vomits or takes laxatives, or both. The bulimic has the "satisfaction" of abnormal ingestion of food and eliminates worry about calories by vomiting it all up.

One similarity between the two disorders is that both the

anorexic and bulimic think about food with every waking hour. Food and eating form an obsession for both. Friends, family, school, recreation, social life take a back seat to food, beautiful (or revolting) food.

"Closet" Ailments

Until a relatively few years ago, anorexia and bulimia were almost ailments-in-the-closet; few people recognized them, let alone sought treatment for the victims. In the last few years, however, magazine articles, television shows and even books have appeared, giving frightening statistics on the problems. Jane E. Brody, writing in a recent issue of the New York *Times*, says of anorexia nervosa:

The problem is said to be epidemic among girls in their late teens (it is estimated that fewer than 10 percent of the cases are male, and only a handful involve women beyond their 20's). Among girls aged 16 to 18, it is estimated, anorexia afflicts one in 250, with some estimates running as high as one in 100. The problem is often precipitated by an emotional crisis, resistance to sexual maturity or response to such an innocent remark as "Your jeans are getting tight." Whatever the trigger, it leads to a diet that soon gets out of hand; diuretics, laxatives or purgatives, and over-zealous exercising may also be resorted to."

Ms. Brody points out that severe effects such as prematurely aging skin, menstrual cessation, personality changes for the worse, and injuries to a variety of internal organs are not unusual. She warns:

"Without proper treatment, up to 20 percent of the victims die from the irreversible effects of chronic starvation. Others are saved by being hospitalized against their wills and force-fed, though their underlying problems may remain. Many eventually outgrow the illness on their own, though often without resolving the conflicts that precipitated it...."

If any of you young adult readers even suspect you might be hooked on either disorder, it's never too late to seek help. Chances are, you can't shake either addiction alone. Besides your family doctor, teacher, professor, or clergyman, there are "eating disorder" clinics throughout the country to help on a confidential basis. Your city or county department of mental health can steer you toward a knowledgeable specialist in or near your neighborhood.

The problem is so serious among young adults that there are a number of centers that can provide further information. These include:

National Association of Anorexia Nervosa and
    Associated Disorders
Box 271
Highland Park, IL 60035

American Anorexia Nervosa Association
133 Cedar Lane
Teaneck, NJ 07666

Anorexia Nervosa and Related Eating Disorders
    (ANRED)
Box 1012
Grover City, CA 63433

C H A P T E R • V I I

Calcium Versus Cholesterol

A family favorite, a then stubborn little girl of divorced parents, was at one time in the care of anxious grandparents, who constantly pressed her to drink gallons of milk so she might "put a little weight on." Sally had a thing about the pale color of the milk and took it upon herself at age ten to boycott the hated "moo juice." She was the middle child, with two brothers who lived with their father and his new wife.

The boys seemed to have near-perfect teeth—two visits a year to the dentist just for cleaning. But by her mid-twenties their sister had lost six molars, two incisors, and two bicuspids.

By then a nurse, Sally knew her nutrition and the importance of calcium to teeth and bones. Her dentist knew her history, but he told her it was too late for milk. Calcium from milk, he was convinced, helped only in the growing and development years. No dummy, he was just parroting the view of the time. Sally once again opposed the establishment. What about, she reasoned to herself, bones getting brittle if they were fed no calcium as the years went on?

By the age of thirty-five, half of Sally's teeth were gone. But Sally, even in shock after each extraction, continued her delayed devotion to milk and dairy products in her daily diet. It worked out, at least for her. A lifelong athlete, she suffered no bone disasters in skating and skiing accidents, no fractured hips, no broken shoulder bones, arms, or legs, no shattered ribs. Now sixty-six years old, "senior citizen" Sally is packing for a two-month trip that includes plans for mountain climbing in Europe.

One case? Yes. Actually, it proves nothing, and it's a tossup whether Sally's stress on calcium foods through her adult life, or her genes, or some other good fairy, is responsible for her sound-bone mountain-climbing at age sixty-six.

But it's one possible argument against those who still believe that milk and milk products and green vegetables are only for babies and toddlers. And Sally's story comes to the front burner when one considers the current calcium-versus-cholesterol controversy.

Here's another true story. A family friend, a swimming champ with a sound grasp of physiology and nutrition, as a young married woman took very seriously the importance of nutrients especially during pregnancy. Once the obstetrician had made a positive diagnosis, Elena (always proud of her smile) substituted milk for tea or coffee at every meal and made sure most of her snacks were cheese and her dinner vegetables mostly dark green and leafy. Not only did she produce three beautiful daughters with strong and sound bone structure, but after the birth of the second daughter she was the puzzled but proud possessor of two "new" wisdom teeth.

Only two cases, not earth-shaking, but they seem worth mentioning.

What *is* calcium, anyway?

Calcium is a mineral (like ore or sand but in crystalline form), in color a silvery white, in composition a soft metallic chemical (as in limestone).

Important to us and our diet is the fact that calcium is the most abundant mineral element in the human body. It is half of a team with phosphorus (a nonmetallic element) that is responsible for the hardness of the teeth and bones. About 99 percent of the body's calcium is in tissue of bones and teeth.

The body is miserly with its use of calcium, doling out a tiny amount to other body tissues to help with the balanced performance of heart, nerves, and muscles. A most vital ability of calcium is its help in coagulating (clotting) the blood.

The skeleton, or bony framework, contains just about all of the physical storage places of calcium. The body of an average-sized young adult contains about 1,200 grams (about seven ounces) of calcium, a small fraction of his or her body weight. Of this, 99 percent is deposited in bone as a phosphorus-containing compound.

The calcium and phosphate molecules (particles) in the bone do not stay static for a person's lifetime; from time to time they are replaced in bodily exchange by new molecules. Just a theory right now, it is believed that a few grams of calcium in the young adult or adult are on a kind of daily merry-go-round in this way.

The bottom line seems to be that the body desperately needs calcium, not only during babyhood and the growing years, but every day in life. If some calcium is not taken in daily, as a defense and life-saving mechanism, the body has no choice but to steal it from the storage places in the bones. As a chronic and sustained process, this can and will make the bones lose their strength and density, their ability to withstand cracks and fractures.

Enter the Villain

Cholesterol is a word that has come into layman's language only in the last few years. It's not easy to spell or understand, but it has been familiar to the medical community for many decades.

Let's see where it comes from. The word is derived from *chol-*, a Greek prefix meaning "gall," plus *stereos*, meaning "solid." Put them together and you have "solid gall" or "hard mass."

Cholesterol is a fatty substance normally manufactured in all living tissues, including those of the human body, and basic to health and the body's operation. So the body gets it in two ways: by manufacturing it and by ingesting it in the daily diet. If too much cholesterol gets into the bloodstream, however, it can build up on the walls of the arteries, narrowing the passageways of the blood in its circulation and setting the stage for heart attack and stroke.

A fatty gruellike substance, cholesterol is a very complex steroid (solid and ringed) alcoholic substance. Under the microscope it shows itself in greasy yellow-white crystals; these crystals do not dissolve in water, although sometimes they can be diluted in other fats, ether (the compound like the anesthetic), or simpler alcohol forms.

As far as is known, cholesterol seems to share some of the basic characteristics of simple fats. Like other components of fats, it goes through a number of chemical changes as the body readies it for use. One of the changes is into *cholesterol ester* (an *ester* is a compound formed from the combination of an alcohol and an acid), which occurs when the cholesterol abandons its end-alcohol group of components and picks up a kind of fatty acid.

Cholesterol, in short, is nothing new. It's as old as mankind, and perhaps older. It's a chemical component of all animal oils and fats.

A little cholesterol, the amount normally manufactured for its own use by the body, is a good thing. It's of vital importance to the process of metabolism. It's like your mom making a pie crust "from scratch" using basic ingredients. A well-balanced measure of certain ingredients means a smooth, flaky crust. Too much shortening or lard or baking powder means a tough hard mess—like too much cholesterol from the bloodstream clinging to the walls of the arteries to dam up the circulation.

The Battle of the Bulge

It was bad timing when opposing arguments surfaced in the same recent decades in the world of medical information.

As noted, the medical community learned that calcium was a vital nutrient: not confined to baby nourishment, but needed throughout life. People began to read more and more about the theory that bones lose their density and strength, at any age, when deprived of dietary calcium. As a matter of fact, the longer we live, the more brazen the body becomes in its theft of calcium from the bones.

Then there surfaced the two great warring factions on cholesterol. One says, and remains convinced, that the cholesterol found in certain foods, particularly "saturated" fats, was the major villain in the buildup of cholesterol in the bloodstream and on the walls of the arteries.

The other says that the accusation against cholesterol-containing foods is nonsense, or at least badly exaggerated.

By the second half of this century, the battle was joined. On the whole, it made pretty good newspaper and magazine copy, reporting successes or failures for each side. Top reporters of the war were the New York *Times*, the Washington *Post*, *Time* magazine, and other print media of that stature. Top generals in the debate were the likes of the American Heart Association, the National Institutes of Health, and the National Research Council. The ground troops were made up of small cadres of physiologists, nutritionists, and research groups.

One point on which all the experts agreed was that all the "bad" cholesterol buildup had to come from dietary habits. Also agreed on were two relevant factors: calcium was of proven value to nutrition, and evidence was pretty conclusive that too much of "hard fats" in the diet contributed to cholesterol buildup in the blood and the arteries.

You may have a friend or relative whose bones break easily from minor falls or accidents. That can happen for a number of reasons, but many such mishaps are due to the fact that the victim's bone structure is "undernourished" in its major nutrient support—calcium.

The U.S. Nutrition Foundation in Washington, D.C.,

which records such figures, reported recently that osteoporosis, a deteriorative condition, disables about 14 million women in the United States.

The broken hip, we must admit, is frequent among senior citizens, mostly women. It happens most often to women after menopause, but it can and does happen to those much younger, the young adult age group for example.

People serious about trying for a long and healthy life began to question the conflicting warnings to maintain the calcium level and at the same time keep down the sludge or cholesterol in their bodies, which made no sense. If milk, cheese, and other dairy products were their best source of bone-protecting calcium, how about the fat in those foods that would at the same time pile on the cholesterol? And what about those with some kind of allergy to the milk group?

Not to worry. There is at least a partial answer, though it isn't a simple one. We've already learned that it's possible to avoid whole milk without avoiding calcium. Low-fat, skim, or powdered milk contains just about as much calcium as whole milk, without the generous supply of fat; and low-fat yogurt (try it!) is said to have more calcium than fat-containing cheeses.

Are you allergic to milk? It's a condition called lactose intolerance. Ask your doctor about calcium supplements. He'll recommend, if he thinks you need it, calcium carbonate. Good brands are available on the commercial/pharmaceutical market. But use the product strictly as the doctor prescribes; overdoses can be toxic.

Remember also that milk isn't the sole source of calcium. Among green vegetables extra generous with their calcium gifts are collard, turnip, and mustard greens.

Certain members of the fish family have other virtues than the fact that they make good (and tasty) substitutes for red meat. Sardines and their bones (packed and canned in water), oysters, and salmon are top sources of calcium.

One Man's Meat

Speaking of meat substitutes, Americans have a reputation for being the heartiest meat-eaters in the world. Many pediatricians believe that parents start meat too soon in their baby foods; maybe that is where the meat hang-up gets started. The basic nutrient of meat as a foodstuff is the protein. The baby doctors believe that most infants get more than enough protein in their milk and eggs.

Anxious parents and grandparents believe to this day that all growing children must have at least three servings of meat daily. Not true. The result of too much meat fed to the small fry can be "protein poisioning," an imbalance in types of nutrition.

It wasn't always so. Time was when few Americans were beefeaters. Until well into this century, Americans had little taste for beef. What was available came from cattle that "roamed the range"; they ate what they found when they found it, and their meat had little fat and was tough, gamy, and stringy.

Then, as cattle-raising became refined and more sophisticated, the toughness was tenderized and "prime" beef came from steers or domestic bulls fed on corn. The red meat was now tender and more tasty because it was "marbled" (veined) with hard and saturated fat.

Score one more for those arguing the higher cholesterol content of red meats.

CHAPTER • VIII

Vitamins and Vitality

What are vitamins? And what do they have to do with the whole nutrition scene?

First, here's what they're not, much of that having to do with popular misunderstanding.

When vitamins are mentioned or advertised (as they are with a vengeance), most people think of them as a sort of medicinal pill, a substitute for food that takes the place of having to eat.

Not so. Vitamins are tiny components of food, but they're not food, as such. They're no substitute for carbohydrates and minerals and proteins and fats and water. The body doesn't manufacture vitamins; they must be taken in with the food we eat and the water and liquids we drink.

Vitamins are *catalysts* (changers), materials or chemical agents that act to cause or promote other chemical activities or reactions or changes in the body and its metabolic function. Vitamins, as part of the food we eat, help the body to utilize other nutrients that are taken into the body in the eating process. But even though they're very important, it is said that all thirteen vitamins needed in the daily diet are needed in such small amounts that the total could fit into an eighth of a teaspoon.

The whole story of vitamins and our knowledge of them began in the early seventeenth century when British navy officers began to give their sailors fruit juice as part of their daily grub without really knowing why. They had simply noticed that the fruit juice seemed to ward off deadly diseases such as scurvy and beri-beri during long sea voyages.

By the nineteenth century, chemists in several countries undertook serious research on why certain types of food fought certain diseases.

In 1912 a Polish chemist named Casimir Funk came up with the idea that a chemical compound called an *amine* and its family of related compounds were so vital to human nourishment that a lack of any of them could bring on one of the fatal diseases.

He suggested calling that family of amines something like *vitamines*—*vita*, the Latin word for "life," and *amines* for the chemical compounds. In later years the final *e* was dropped, and we have the modern name *vitamins*.

Today we know the vitamins as supplements to the diet, to be taken in commercial tablet or liquid *only* as prescribed by the physician.

Nutritionists tell us that the odds are strong against the average teenager or young adult needing vitamin supplements, unless the doctor discovers through clinical tests a serious lack of a certain vitamin in the chemical makeup. Unless he or she lives mainly on junk, all the vitamins needed are supplied through breakfast, lunch, dinner, and in-between snacks.

What happens if we goof somehow on vitamin intake? A temporary shortage of one or more kinds of vitamins isn't too serious, in the short run, while you're young. But the shortage, kept up over an extended period of time, can mean poor nourishment of the veins and arteries, bringing on arteriosclerosis (hardening of the arteries) or weakening of the heart muscle (heart disease). It can contribute toward the shortening of one's life.

Maybe you think your high school chemistry course is or was gross, a dull drag. Don't knock it too much.

It probably emphasized for you that all living things, to

keep on living and growing, must have a constant supply of *chemical energy*. All animals—including human animals between the ages of twelve and twenty—get that chemical energy from the food they eat. In all forms of life, the energy is released for use when the food (in the form that cells can use) is oxidized (combined with the oxygen that is supplied by fresh air).

Foods themselves are made up of one or more chemical compounds that cells use for assimilation (absorption into the system for nourishment), growth (of the body and its organs), and cell repair.

These compounds, known as *nutrients*, consist of such basic substances as carbohydrates, fats proteins, and vitamins, which are in the category of *organic compounds*. The *inorganic compounds* are water and mineral salts, which complete the list of ingested items that are necessary to life and growth.

So you see, the whole "extended family" of vitamins makes up only one type of element that you need for nutrition during your young adult years.

Consumer groups continue to be disturbed by what they consider the outright shafting of the public in the promotion of vitamins. Commercialization, competition, and promotion seem to them aimed to lay a guilt trip on all of us who do not spend big bucks to stuff ourselves with all kinds of vitamins.

It is believed that this is true among the more vulnerable late teens who occasionally haunt the health food stores and their vitamin displays almost as they would the record-and-tape section of the local department store.

Vitamins and what they do to keep us going isn't easy to understand. They can't give us energy, pep, vim and vigor in a direct way, but we've got to have them, in the right amounts, so that the body cells can carry out their proper functions.

As we've seen, some vitamins help the body make blood cells, hormones (chemical products produced by a gland), and other regulating substances you need day and night, waking and sleeping. Other types of vitamins make possible better use of other nutrients.

Know Your Alphabet

We're told that thirteen vitamins are necessary for sound health. Four of them are known as fat-soluble vitamins because they literally dissolve in fat. Vitamins A, D, E, and K are digested or assimilated (absorbed) with the help of fats in the diet.

These four vitamins can be stored in the body for relatively long periods of time, mainly in the fatty tissues and the liver. Thus it is not necessary to eat food rich in those vitamins every day.

The other nine vitamins are called water-soluble: eight from the B vitamin family and vitamin C. Because they cannot be stored in the body for long, the daily diet should include foods that are rich sources of these vitamins.

In that alphabet caper, here's a rundown on the main vitamins and what they do for you:

Vitamin A. It is necessary to good eyesight, good skin, strong bones, and the healing of cuts and bruises as well as more serious wounds. Vitamin A is contained in fruits and vegetables, fish, milk and milk products, and liver.

Vitamin(s) B. In the family of B vitamins, various ones launch the body's proper use of protein, fats, and carbohydrates; some help trigger the work of the brain and the nervous system. B vitamins are contained in many foods such as whole-grain and enriched cereals and breads, meats, and beans.

Vitamin C. It helps in the healing of bruises and abrasions, promotes the building of blood vessels, nourishes teeth, bones, and all kinds of tissue, and works with minerals used by the body. Vitamin C is found mainly in citrus fruits, melons, berries, and leafy green vegetables including broccoli, spinach, and cabbage.

Vitamin D. It enables the body to utilize calcium and phosphorus, which build strong bones and teeth. (Your skin gets the advantages of vitamin D when it enjoys a mild amount of sunshine.) Vitamin D is found in fish, liver, and eggs and is added commercially to milk.

Vitamin E. It is believed that it promotes the health of cell tissues. Vitamin E is found in many foods, but the best sources are vegetable oils and whole-grain cereals.

Vitamin K. It has to do with the normal clotting of the blood. (When you've had cuts on your skin, you've seen the blood congeal—clot—over the wound, stopping the bleeding.) We get Vitamin K mostly in dark green vegetables, peas, cauliflower, and whole grains. It is also manufactured in the body.

Another family of nutrients might be called second cousins to the vitamins: They are minerals and trace elements. *Trace* describes minerals that we need in daily nutrition in very tiny amounts—a few millionths of an ounce: iron, copper, zinc, and others.

Once again, don't waste your money on the advertising hype of vitamin manufacturers. With a balanced diet, you get all the vitamins you need; the added pills are nothing but waste. Don't be a vitamin pill popper as if they're going out of style. They're not—not while the XYZ Vitamin Company is showing a big profit from your loyalty.

Recently doctors and nutritionists have been trying to get across to the public, of all ages, that it's possible to get too much of a good thing with certain vitamins. Some of them can be toxic, seriously poisonous, in careless overdose.

For example, the body needs such tiny amounts of vitamins A, D, and K and iron that a little too much can mean a lot too much. "A little too much" of A and D and the trace elements can undermine one's general health. An oversupply of iron in the body can seriously damage certain organs. Too much of the B's can cancel out their normal benefits and make unreasonable demands of other vitamins.

Some nutritionists tell us to beware of minerals in general; overdoses of phosphorus, calcium, and magnesium can so upset the body's natural chemistry that actual bone loss could take place.

It goes without saying that excesses can be even worse for children, teenagers, and young adults who are still growing and don't yet have the natural protections that come with full-grown adulthood.

The best authorities agree on this bottom line. The average person, including the young adult, who suffers from vitamin deficiency actually suffers from a dumb choice of nonnourishing foods.

Since the days of Casimir Funk, research on vitamins has been accepted, speeded up, added to, and has met with all kinds of controversy, in this country and internationally. It ranges from the assertion that "nobody needs to take vitamins" to many hucksters who claim that "nobody takes enough vitamins."

It is generally agreed that the average young adult can get all of his or her nutrients, including vitamins, from a balanced diet; vitamins from pills and liquids, as far as we know, are at best only nutrition supplements and should be taken under a doctor's direction and supervision.

Energy Engineering

A young lady of our acquaintance, a pretty eighteen-year-old, was coming down the home stretch in her freshman year at college. We asked her from time to time how she liked the first rung of climbing the collegiate ladder. Besides the usual "School is school," we often got "I'm always so tired, I actually fall asleep in class. Guess I'm bored."

Her bag is science, and we could sympathize about compulsory attendance at the "liberal arts" and literature courses. That wasn't the whole story, however; a closer look at her nutrition life-style gave a better clue to her constant fatigue.

Donna admitted that she had early classes and "no time at all for breakfast." She worked in the school library during the lunch break, at which time she usually had a Coke and a bag of potato chips. Dinner was a sometime thing, mostly when her parents took her to a restaurant; when she was alone at home, "dinner" was a handful of chocolate chip cookies.

Although tiny and slim, obviously she wasn't putting enough unleaded fuel in the small sports-car tank she called her body, so it was running below par. She summed it up herself: She had "absolutely no energy."

Fashionable as her pencil-slim figure might be, it basically was lacking calories: units of heat supplied by food for energy.

What has energy to do with food? Literally, "energy" means "capacity for vigorous activity." Donna's physical activity wasn't vigorous. It didn't exist. That meant she had less physical clout than she should, not only for philosophy and English Lit. but for the discotheque and tennis court as well.

Donna and everyone in the young adult age group need more, not less, of the energy builders in the daily diet. All of them are individuals, of course, but at least some of them are still "growing" and developing, and the growth process is in effect stealing from the pep-giving foods they eat.

There's a smidgen of truth in claims for the commercially advertised candy bar: It does produce a supply of quick (though temporary) energy. The average candy bar contains 150 calories, basically supplied by the ingredients of sugar. Sugar is actually a group of carbohydrates that the body digests and uses easily and quickly. It is famous (or notorious) for satisfying sudden pangs of hunger. But you can get that sugar sensation from snacks like raisins and raw prunes without endangering your tooth enamel.

Used as a sweetener, "table sugar" is a concentrated form of calories, or energy. A tablespoon of sugar (about one-half ounce) yields 60 calories, or units of heat that the body uses in energy output. The refined sugar people use in tea or coffee or sprinkle over that tart grapefruit isn't the only kind. Some 5 percent of cow's milk is lactose or "milk sugar." Some fruits contain fruit sugar, which is also found in concentrated amounts in dried fruits such as raisins, figs, and prunes.

We must remember that the sources of "sugar" as such make up only one type of nutrient that the body needs. Sugar gets attention here because teens and young adults tend to go overboard on calories and the danger of overweight because of a "sweet tooth."

The experts tell us that at least fifty types of nutrients are vital to growth, development, and health of the body. Leave out one, even by accident, and you're missing a link in the nutrition chain. Even one link in the long chain can be serious.

Probably holding top rank in qualifying for energy supply are fats and carbohydrates. All fats are pretty much macho in this department; they supply a large amount of energy in comparison to the relatively small serving size of the food item. Some nutritionists believe that only 35 percent or less of a daily diet should be fats. The best sources of fat are oil, shortening, butter (or margarine), such meats as bacon, fat on other meats, chocolate, and nuts.

The carbohydrates we eat supply immediate energy and help the body make the best use of other nutrients. Carbohydrates are obtained mainly from cereals, various sugars and ingredients of "sweets," pastas (the spaghetti family), fresh fruits such as bananas, dried fruits, and vegetables such as lima beans, corn, and potatoes.

The fats and carbohydrates are only two of the "energy" nutrients. Others of major importance and their sources include:

Nutrient	Sources
PROTEIN: Builds, repairs, and regulates body tissues; forms antibodies to fight infection.	Meats, fish, poultry, dried beans and peas, milk and milk products, nuts and nut products such as peanut butter.
CALCIUM: Essential in building strong bones and teeth from birth to adulthood and beyond; activates enzymes (the body's "converters"), which change food into energy.	Milk, milk products (especially cheese), sardines, shellfish, all green leafy vegetables, turnips.
PHOSPHORUS: Like milk, helps to build and preserve teeth and bones; necessary to certain enzymes in converting food into energy.	Fish, meat, poultry, dried peas and beans, milk and milk products, egg yolk; whole-grain cereals and breads.
IRON: Works with protein to manufacture hemoglobin (the red blood cells), which transports oxygen from lungs to cells; helps to store oxygen in muscle; fights anemia.	Liver, red meat, shellfish, eggs, dark green vegetables, peas and beans, dried fruits like apricots, prunes, raisins; whole-grain bread and cereal; molasses.
IODINE: Vital to good performance of the thyroid gland, which secretes a hormone that regulates the body's growth and development; fights goiter.	Seafood; iodized (fortified with iodine, a chemical found in seawater) table salt.

Nutrient	Sources
THIAMIN (also called vitamin B₁): improves appetite and digestion, aids the nervous system, necessary for certain enzymes that change food into energy.	Meat, especially pork and liver, dried peas and beans, whole-grain and enriched breads and cereals, wheat germ.
RIBOFLAVIN (also called vitamin B₂): Aids the cells in use of oxygen; vital to good eyesight and skin; also needed for certain enzymes that convert food to energy.	Milk and milk products (especially cheese), liver, green leafy vegetables, meat, eggs, enriched breads and cereals.
NIACIN (also called nicotinic acid): Good for normal appetite, proper digestion, healthy nervous system; also needed to help enzymes convert food into energy.	Liver, meat, fish, poultry, green vegetables, peanuts, whole-grain and enriched breads and cereals.

The following vitamins are also essential, particularly for the young adult who is still growing and developing:

Vitamin	Sources
VITAMIN C (also called ascorbic acid): Helps keep cells adhering together; toughens walls of blood vessels; aids healthy gums; helps fight infection, promote healing.	Citrus fruits; certain vegetables, especially broccoli, cabbage, cauliflower, and potatoes; "summer fruits" such as strawberries and melons.
VITAMIN A: Helps keep skin and eyesight in healthful state; needed for growth, development, and resisting infection.	Liver, fish liver oils, dark green vegetables and deep yellow fruits and vegetables, eggs, butter, enriched margarine, and skim milk.
VITAMIN D: Aids the body in utilizing calcium and phosphorus and building bones and teeth.	Fortified milk, fish liver oils, egg yolk.

Other nutrients, some newly recognized, can be considered important for the young adult. These include vitamin B₆, vitamin B₁₂, folic acid (spinach is a great source), vitamin E, vitamin K, and magnesium.

There's the laundry list of things you need in your diet. Although some of the nutrients named have the reputation of being "energy" sources, it's clear that they depend on each other and must work together to keep the machine of the body well oiled and tuned.

What's more, they depend practically without exception on the work of the enzyme, the special kind of protein manufactured by the body to speed the breakdown of complex substances in food.

Let's go back to the two particular kinds of nutrients associated with quick energy fats and carbohydrates.

Our most compact and concentrated form of energy is *fats*. By comparison, an ounce of fat has about double the number of calories as the same amount of either protein or carbohydrate.

Fats supply the calories and also have the job of transporting four important vitamins throughout the body (the "fat-soluble" vitamins).

Two important characteristics of fats affect nourishment for the young adult and to a certain extent for those in other age groups. Basically, fat for most people is out-and-out fattening. It is in concentrated amounts in your favorite snacks: potato chips, french fries, deep-fried hamburgers, "frosted" dry cereals, and heavy salad dressings. No doubt about it, stuffing yourself constantly with them will make you fat.

At your age as well as in later years, nutritionists believe, most Americans eat too much fat. As we grow older, eating too much fat makes us easy marks for such life-threatening diseases as high blood pressure, heart disease, stroke, and even cancer.

Carbohydrates and fats have about the same prime power to supply energy. They are not identical, however, and they have different side effects and different after effects in the process of nourishment.

Actually, there are three kinds of *carbohydrates*.

Simple carbohydrates, what we think of as real sugars, are found in fruits, milk, and even some vegetables such as beets and peas. Refined (cultivated or processed) sugars from such plants as cane sugar and sugar beets are mainly used as additives to sweets of all kinds—candy, cake, soft drinks, ice cream.

Starch, another type of multicomposition carbohydrate, is found in bread, potatoes, some vegetables, and rice. **Fiber**, a third type, is part of the walls of plant cells. Tough or stringy, it is found in the bran of wheat and other cereals and can be seen and tasted in raw celery. In the process of nutrition, here's how it all works. When carbohydrates are introduced into your body, starches and sugars are changed to *glucose*, a substance manufactured by the body that enables it to assimilate the carbohydrates. Glucose is a basic fuel for the cell, producing energy and heat.

When the body receives more carbohydrates than it needs at a given time, some is converted into *glycogen*, which the body then stores. If in emergency the body needs an extra spurt of energy, the glycogen is converted back into glucose to be used directly for energy. The rest of the "energy chemical" is stored as fat—really solid storage for the future.

Carbohydrates and fats are necessary to keep the body mechanism running like fine clockwork, but they can be too much of a good thing. At the risk of sounding like a broken record, they must be taken in proper amounts.

Only the "balanced diet" and daily "balanced menu" can act like a computer to allot the right amounts: now as a builder, and later to maintain a sound adulthood and act as a strong force in delaying the signs of old age.

Serving by Serving ... Foods Provide for Daily Needs*

Stars on the chart below give a general idea of how servings of familiar foods contribute toward dietary needs—the more stars, the better the food as a source of the nutrient. The percentages given below the chart are based on the National Research Council's recommended dietary allowances for a man. For some kinds of food, values are for a specific food. For others, values are for a food group; in a varied diet, which is common in this country, group values are likely to average as shown.

Kind of food	Size of Serving	Iron	Calcium	Protein	B-vitamins	Vitamin A value	Thiamin	Riboflavin	Vitamin C (ascorbic acid)	Food energy (in calories)
Milk, whole fluid	1 cup	*	****		*			***		160
Cheese, process Cheddar	1 ounce	*	***		*			*		115
Meat, poultry, fish (lean)	2 ounces	***		**	*	*		*		140
Eggs	1 large	*		*	*			*		80
Dry beans	¾ cup	**	*	****		*		*		160
Peanut butter	2 tbsp.	*		*						190
Bread, whole wheat	2 slices	*	*	**			*			135
Bread, enriched	2 slices	*		*			*	*		135
Cereal, ready-to-eat	1 ounce			***	**	**	**		**	110
Citrus juice	½ cup					*			*****	50
Other fruit, fruit juice	½ cup			*	*				***	80
Tomatoes, tomato juice	½ cup			*	**	*			*****	30
Dark-green and deep-yellow vegetables	½ cup		*	*	*****			*	****	45
Potatoes	1 medium			*			*		****	75
Other vegetables	½ cup			*	*				**	30
Butter, margarine	1 tbsp.					*				100
Sugar	2 teaspoons									25
Molasses	2 tbsp.	**	****							95

Part of daily need from a serving:
*****About 50 percent or more.
****About 40 percent.

***About 30 percent.
**About 20 percent.
*About 10 percent.

*SOURCE: *Nutrition Food At Work For You.* Published by the Prudential Insurance Company of America, with cooperation of the United States Department of Agriculture.

Rip-off Trio:
Health, Organic, Natural

Who are the shahs of shafting when it comes to false claims of nutrition for their foods? If you say McDonald's or Burger King or Chicken Delight, think again. You're dead wrong.

While our Crew of Cooks mainly take advantage of the middle-aged and oldsters, the young adult world is increasingly becoming vulnerable to invasion. Promoters are going more after young people, no doubt because their income in allowances and baby-sitting fees is looking up; now there's cash for the taking among them. Youthful idealism and the fitness craze add to their gullibility for the brazen claims for "health" foods and "organic" or "natural" foods.

One menacing minus must be scored against the pluses chalked up by nutrition education in high school and college. That is the possibility of the young people's getting so fired up by ideas about proper food, balanced diet, and maximum nutrition that they frequent the "health food store" about as much as their misguided parents or grandparents.

For starters, "health" foods, "organic" foods, and "natural" foods have one thing in common: They cost a lot. Sometimes they cost much more than the conventionally grown and manufactured products (with all their evil contents of additives, fertilizers, and pesticides).

There's an old saying that the higher the price, the easier it is to bamboozle the American purchaser, regardless of age.

Maybe so. Look at the cosmetics industry. Most women (and men) seem to prefer to pay $50 for a highly advertised "wrinkle remover" rather than use a cheap household product such as petroleum jelly, baby oil, or vegetable oil that may provide the same protection and softening for the skin and in many cases, better.

The same goes for food products. If we pay $2.59 for a box of cereal at the health food store, it's bound to give us more and purer nutrition than the $1.69 item at the supermarket.

Not so. Sez who? For one, the U.S. Department of Agriculture, which has done extensive research over the past few years and has concluded that "organic" and "nonorganic" foods are equal in nutrient quality.

What's the real meaning of those magic words that mean super sales and profits? Webster tells us that "health" is the "condition of being sound in body, mind or spirit." Will it make you unsound physically, mentally, or spiritually if your mom serves a can of beans without the health-food label? Nonsense.

Webster defines "organic" as "relating to or produced without the use of chemically formulated fertilizer and pesticide." What are your odds on surviving if you eat apples grown in soil treated with fertilizer? "Natural," Noah has been sure for decades, is "being in accordance with or determined by nature." That commercial-brand slice of cheese may be "unnatural" only if you're hungry and somehow can't get your hands on it.

But according to the health-food store owner or salesman, all three words are synonymous. They are not, by any means. Lumping them together doesn't make them identical, but it does give promoters more leeway and extra words or phrases to help push their over-priced wares.

It doesn't happen often, but the author has seen shoppers at the supermarket who scan labels for that magic phrase "natural ingredients." If a label admits to the content of sugar, salt, artificial coloring, preservatives, or additives, the can or package is promptly put back on the shelf with a shudder of revolt.

A man of our acquaintance, in his late 70's, walks half a mile to his "health food store" to stock up on cereal, honey, wheat germ oil, sunflower seeds, and many other "organic" items, some of them higher priced or even double the price of the same goodies in the supermarket a block from his house.

This fall guy isn't a young adult, and he's not stupid. He's a retired engineer with all the proper academic credentials. But he's a sitting duck for the health-food fairy tales he reads in newspaper and magazine advertisements.

Swear Words: Pesticides and Fertilizers

"Additives" and "artificial coloring" and "preservatives" are no-no's among the health-food faddists. The big curse words are "pesticide" and "fertilizers." If the food product doesn't boast innocence of having been grown and processed without either one of the two, it is an admission of poison. Let's glance at the development of both.

Our great-great grandparents, and further back, worked long and weary hours to get enough food from the soil to feed their families. By today's standards and methods, the work was so demanding and frustrating in all probability because the time had not come for the use of pesticides and fertilizers.

The average young adult, without knowing the facts, may imagine that in the growing and processing his hamburger, his peas and carrots, his mashed potatoes were generously sprinkled with deadly chemical sprays.

Not so. Years ago, the modern chemical methods employed to improve and revitalize the soil and kill the pests that would otherwise ruin the food were placed under federal regulation.

Pure food laws have long been adopted to police the farming, growing, and processing of all foods to retain only the tiniest trace of pesticides. Doctors Victor Herbert and Stephen Barrett point out, in their book *Vitamins and Health Foods—The Great American Hustle*:

There has not been one case of illness in America which can be attributed to a scientific agricultural procedure. In contrast, in countries where "organic" fertilizers (such as human waste) are used food poisoning from disease organisms is quite common.

It would be foolish to claim that "organic foods" are harmful or nonbeneficial. But some doctors have asserted that patients who confine their food purchases to the high-priced stores often lack significant amounts of such nutrients as protein and carbohydrates that they need for optimum health.

Again, the bottom line in describing the health food store is *expensive*. Plenty of Americans today, including the young adult who takes an occasional food shopping trip, consider the prices at the supermarket high enough. They see no "shrinking inflation" when it comes to pantry and breadbox items.

Bright young adults on the whole are unlikely to go the extra mile to pay for overpriced items in the health food store. They leave that to people like my elderly engineer friend. But that has a sad note. Doctors are concerned about senior citizens on fixed incomes being taken in by ads and fliers with extravagant (and untrue) claims for the users.

You're much too young to remember the colorful period of American history called the "snake-oil era." That was the time, about a century ago, when clever and money-hungry pitchmen operated from horse-drawn wagons, stopping here and there across the country to sell their concoctions that were supposed to guarantee long life, supreme health, and cures for all sorts of ills: arthritis, gout, chronic fatigue, pimples, wrinkles, freckles, and poor sexual performance. These magic lotions were usually brownish liquids and were known to the wary as "snake oil."

Again, the health food store does not purvey poison. The average health food store is at worst a gyp joint. Its salesmen and promoters abuse their faithful clientele by the simple scheme of overcharging. "Freedom of speech" and "freedom of the press" keep them out of jail. The promoters, many nutritionists believe, are for the most part food faddists. A few sincerely believe in the junk they peddle, but most are interested solely in one product—greenbacks.

Bites on a Budget

Maybe you've reached that magic "independent" age of eighteen. You're living in your own apartment alone or with a roommate. Or for one reason or other, you're already picking up the tab for the necessities of life.

Chances are that when you first struck out on your own, your biggest shock came with the quotation of monthly rent. Horrendous! But no getting around it, you needed a roof over your head.

Unless you're a slave to fashion and clothes, the next shock was the cost of food for that table you planned to bum from Mom's cellar or Aunt Kate's attic.

No fooling around with the food any more. Junk food had to be out. No more tasty but expensive bags of potato chips, if you were paying. Maybe you've learned a little about nutrition and you won't waste your precious cash, wherever you get it, on empty calories in your menu.

It could be that you're bored stiff with the "Basic Four" theory you've heard in school, but the theory can trigger a good start on a relatively simple food-purchase plan. And you can work out such a plan with the greatest of ease.

The U.S. Department of Agriculture has developed the "Daily Food Guide" of Basic-Four types of food to ease the burden for the one who takes charge of the food shopping. Here's the list of basic food needs by category:

Milk Group
2 servings per day for adults
4 servings: teenagers
3 servings: children
Foods made from milk contribute part of the nutrients supplied by a serving of milk.

Meat Group
2 servings
Dry beans and peas, soy extenders, and nuts combined with animal protein (meat, fish, poultry, eggs, milk, cheese) or grain protein can be substituted for a serving of meat.

Fruit-Vegetable Group
4 servings
Dark green leafy or orange vegetables and fruit are recommended three or four times weekly. Citrus fruit (oranges, lemons, limes, grapefruit) is recommended daily.

Cereal Group
4 servings
Whole grain, fortified, or enriched grain products are recommended.

Other
Fats, oils, and sweets complement but do not replace foods from the Basic Four groups. Amounts should be determined by individual caloric needs.

For your young adult age group, it's a cinch that food shopping won't be first priority on your agenda. But if you care at all about sound nourishment and are responsible for what's in the fridge and the pantry—and want to or are forced to watch your pennies—it's a good idea to keep an eye on the Basic Four. For instance, you could type or write a list of the four and tape it on the door of the refrigerator.

Let's talk a little about the foods in each group and how buying habits can save you money.

Milk and Milk Products

Milk is your best source of calcium, that all-important mineral nutrient, and next best are the products using milk as a base. Of course, the fresher, the better. With daily products you can check just how fresh they are by watching the dates on the cartons. There's a law about dating. True, there is such a thing as predating by a distributor. But certainly, if the date on the carton has passed, it's a no-no.

Incidentally, you buy good things like calcium and phosphorus no matter what form of milk you buy. Nutrition experts say that eight ounces of skim milk contains more calcium than eight ounces of whole milk (with all its fat content), and the skim milk is usually cheaper.

Speaking of milk products, try yogurt for variety. Yogurt is made from milk and buttermilk. It's high in calcium, potassium, and phosphorus. For most young people, it's an acquired taste, and it may take a little time for you to become a fan. The yogurts with fruit or fruit flavor are tastier. Nutritionists say that, calorie for calorie, the low-fat brand of yogurt is a better source of calcium than some fat-filled cheeses.

If you're a milk freak, buy it by the gallon; it's cheaper than the one-quart container, and it should keep a week or more.

Back to cheese, which is also in the milk category. It's not true that the more expensive the cheese, the better it is for you. Highest by milligrams in calcium, phosphorus, and vitamin A value, and relatively cheap, is the humble Parmesan cheese used so lavishly in pasta dishes. Less nutritious are the far more expensive blue cheese and Camembert.

Cottage cheese is lower in calories than American or cheddar, but it has all the nutrients. Try Edam or Gouda (not too expensive) to put a little variety in your cheese.

Unless you have a serious weight problem, ice cream is a good bet for occasional snacks or desserts. Like Parmesan, it gets really high marks for calcium, phosphorus, and vitamin A.

Meat Group

For the healthy young adult, nourishing meats include beef, lamb, pork, liver, heart, and kidneys. Not strictly meats, but in that category of nourishment, are poultry and eggs, fish and shellfish.

Alternate items offering the same or similar nutrients include dry beans and peas, lentils, nuts, peanuts (the dry, unsalted ones are best), and peanut butter.

Chosen daily should be two or more servings: a "serving" is two or three ounces of lean cooked meat, poultry, or fish. Fresh fish is best, but it's often hard to find and is more expensive than frozen varieties.

Not keen on either meat or fish? Nutritionists report that two tablespoons of peanut butter can replace in nourishment one-half a serving of meat.

Purchasing hints: Buy the cheapest cuts of meat; avoid veal and lamb chops when their prices are out of sight. In buying fish, avoid the luxury items like shrimp and lobster, both of which are also costly in calories and cholesterol.

You can't beat lentils and a good brand of lentil soup for a combination of nourishment and economy. Keep stocked up on peanut butter, especially when a sale price is involved. Be sensible when storing up your nuts like a squirrel—dry, roasted (unsalted) peanuts for your slim wallet and less salt; pass up such luxuries as the glamorously advertised macadamia nuts (a 3½ ounce jar in some stores is $2.79!), an overpriced item with little nutrition.

Buy meats with as little fat as possible. You're sure to go for hamburger at times; ask your friendly neighborhood butcher to chop the meat fresh and not lard it with a lot of fat.

At the same time, don't make a court case of avoiding *all* fats. In the first place, it's impossible. Besides, fats are "quick energy" foods usually best achieved in meats and dairy foods. The "stored fat" that the body doesn't use immediately isn't just that ugly rubber tire around the waist; at least some of it gives the bony skeleton a certain amount of padding and protection.

Fruit–Vegetable Group

As you might figure, this group includes vegetables and fruits of all kinds, which gives us a wide range in choice and variety.

Compared to the sterling nutritive qualities of milk, nutritionists consider fruits and vegetables equal, or at least numbers two and three, on the staff-of-life list.

Charts of the essential nutrients contained in specific fruits and vegetables give high ranking to many of them, especially in supplying generous amounts of vitamins A and C, of prime importance to the young adult.

For those two vitamins, and other vitamins and nutrients (calcium, phosphorus, protein, trace minerals), you can't top fruits and vegetables. The bottom line is simply that you get more nutrition dollar-for-dollar when you include them on your grocery list.

Among those most frequently recommended are oranges and grapefruit and their juices, cantaloupes, mangoes, strawberries, broccoli, brussels sprouts, and peppers, both the green and sweet-red varieties. Don't forget raw apples; they're not only nutritious, but they provide a supply of necessary fiber.

Incidentally, don't peel the life out of your fruits. A raw apple is better than applesauce. If you have a choice, eat the whole orange instead of settling for juice. When you carefully peel away those white strings on the orange and its rind, you junk some vitamin C.

With just a slightly lower rating in the nutrient community are honeydew melon and watermelon, tangerines, asparagus, cabbage, watercress, potatoes, tomatoes, and turnip greens. Dark green (like spinach) and deep yellow (like carrots) vegetables are recommended as high in nutrients.

What's more, many of the above and their kin, cooked, supply fiber you need and help avoid the expense of buying laxatives.

Speaking of cooked vegetables, don't overboil and leave all the vitamins and nutrients in the cooking water, then throw the water down the drain.

Better than boiling is steaming vegetables. You can buy a wire-basket-type steamer in the dime store. You just set it in the bottom of a cooking pot, place the washed vegetables in it, and cover the bottom of the pot with water. Steam over the burner for just a few minutes and you keep most of the vitamins and nutrients and enhance the taste as well.

Salads of tasty raw vegetables are super. In comparison to other side dishes, they do some great things for your eating health. They clean your teeth with their strong fiber, give your lower jaw lots of exercise, and retain all the natural nourishment without the middleman of cooking loss.

In the interests of your piggy bank, it's really important to buy your fruits and vegetables as fresh as paint. As they age in the bins at the supermarket, they lose some of their nutritive value, and there you are, short-changed in nutrients and vitamins.

Bread–Cereal Group

If you wear glasses, never leave them at home when you're heading for the store to buy these items.

Breads and cereals, cooked or cold, should always be whole-grain or enriched. They cost no more than the others, but your return in vitamins is on the plus side.

Check the labels and packages to make sure you're not being shafted. Some bread wrappers these days are dated so that you can be sure of freshness.

Want a tasty but cheap snack? Try a slice of fresh bread with a little butter or margarine. Or toast it. Toasting doesn't reduce the calories, but to some young people, it improves taste.

Planning with the above guides should be fun, not work or time-consuming.

You plan school courses and what you're going to wear tomorrow, you budget your time to figure what you can spare for sports, dancing, rap sessions.

If you neglect to plan what you're going to put in that wonderful engine called your body, there's a really weak link in the chain of your planning for sensible growth, energy, and nutrition for full adulthood, middle age, and senior years.

The Tooth, the Whole Tooth

Every morsel of food we eat must pass between two rows of white sentinels that start the process of eating and metabolism, the teeth. For the most part, they have had a very bad press.

Some of you have giggled at the zany antics of bucktoothed Bugs Bunny or frozen at the bloody fangs of Transylvania's vampires. That's not the end of the horror story. There's the agony of toothache and cavities, to say nothing of the dentist bills that come to your parents regularly.

By the time of young adulthood, nature has endowed your mouth with thirty-two "second" teeth. Each type of tooth is shaped and scaled to do a specified job. The incisors and canine teeth, toward the front of the mouth, bite and tear the food. The premolars and molars (behind the incisors) grind the food so that it is ready to mix with the digestive juices and proceed with the metabolism.

Though they vary in size and shape, the four types of teeth are made up of identical parts.

The crown is the part of the tooth that is visible above the gumline. The neck is the part under the gum that joins crown and root. The root secures the tooth firmly in the jawbone to which it is attached. The center of the tooth, the pulp, is made up of blood vessels and nerves.

Dentine is the hard, bonelike envelope that encircles the pulp. On the dentine of the crown is the enamel, a layer of material even harder than bone. The dentine is covered by cement, a substance like a thin layer of bone that helps to hold the root in the socket inside the jawbone.

Incidentally, the supply to the teeth of normal and critical hardening substances is heavily dependent on good supplies of vitamin D, phosphate, and calcium and the foods containing them, especially when the second teeth are developing and growing in strength.

There you have the tooth, the whole tooth, and nothing but the tooth.

But it's not all that simple. The teeth make up a critical part of the mouth—not only for chewing and nourishment, but for the shape of the lower part of the face.

Some of you know relatively young people (twenty to thirty years of age) who have lost their teeth and wear dentures, or false teeth.

Dental authorities observe that "some patients lose their teeth before thirty, and some are buried at eighty with all natural teeth intact." They admit that there is no magic formula to guarantee keeping one's natural teeth. That is governed by genes, inherited traits that cause certain families and family lines to lose teeth in early adult years and others to keep their natural teeth into extreme old age.

Sound evidence shows, however, that proper nutrition received before and at time of birth and on through childhood, adolescence, and adulthood will give us an edge in keeping our second teeth through life into senior years. Again, proper nutrition, as well as proper hygiene and dental care, is critical to the growing, developing, and young adult years.

What your dentist calls "dental caries," your parents may call "decaying teeth" or "cavities." Whatever the term used, it means a dismal scene for you and your smile. As more and more teeth are extracted, so is your power to dazzle members of the opposite sex with a happy grin of welcome.

As far as dental experts have been able to find out, dental

caries (the Latin word for *decay*) usually starts on the tooth's crown or enamel with a tiny collection of bacteria and food. This the body promptly changes into a deadly liquid called lactic acid, a top enemy of teeth.

Although the teeth are made of the body's toughest materials, they are particularly susceptible to lactic acid, which is powerful enough to dissolve the enamel.

When it opens up little pits and rows on the tooth's surface, the lactic acid provides fertile soil for the growth of the bacteria in the softer dentine. There they continue to grow and spread, finally reaching the root canal, and that means real pain.

Remember that bacteria just love infected pulp and teeth; like swamps favoring mosquitoes, the decayed spots offer ideal breeding sites for the bacteria. This massive breeding station not only threatens ruin to the teeth but also can bring on abscesses, shooting pus into the bloodstream and thence all through the body.

Now for the dental hygiene routine. Keeping the teeth clean, brushing them after every meal and every snack, cannot be overemphasized. Many dental researchers believe that just about every kind of food can attack the tooth. Some feel that the greatest enemies are such innocent-sounding items as milk, yogurt, sour cream, and other milk products because of their lactic acid content.

Once more, there's no magic way to assure a healthy mouth with sound teeth that will stay around up to and including old age. The dos and don'ts of a sound balanced diet, however, can give you odds on maintaining a dazzling smile.

CHAPTER • XIII

The Sun and You

As has been said, if you are in your late teens or early adult years, you stand a good chance of improving your life expectancy, which at this writing is an average 67.4 years for men and 74.1 for women.

One big blemish in that rosier picture for you is what damage you may be doing right now to your skin. Poor nutrition and careless hygiene are, of course, very bad. But the Number One enemy, in extreme doses, is the sun. "Extreme doses" means keeping a tan the year round or lying in the hot midday sun for hours at a time whenever you get a chance during the summer.

Dermatologists tell us that unrelieved exposure to the sun, at any age, can trigger and speed up the wrinkled, leathery look of the skin to age thirty-five or forty—instead of seventy or eighty.

Remember that your skin, the largest organ of your body, controls body temperature like an efficient thermostat, as well as controlling the vital protection of your internal organs. It's made up primarily of two main parts.

What we see looking at our hands or face is the *epidermis*, or outer and tougher layer of the skin. Immediately beneath the epidermis is the softer and more complex dermis, in which are embedded hair follicles and roots and the sebaceous (fatty or oily) glands, or groups of living cells. The sebaceous glands lubricate the skin itself, keeping it soft and supple.

Forming a cushion under the dermis is a thin layer of subcutaneous (under the skin) fat. It is the sebaceous glands and the thin layer of fat that are, in composition and teamwork, largely responsible for the "youthful" characteristics of the epidermis. The softness and suppleness, as you well know, don't last forever. But there's no sense in speeding up the process of aging years before it's indicated by deliberately drying up the thin layer of softening fat; and that's just what you do when you lie hour after hour in the ultraviolet rays of the sun.

Of course, everyone's skin is unique. Some skin is more vulnerable or tougher than others. Genes come into play there, inherited characteristics that strengthen or weaken the skin, handed down from our parents or grandparents.

For every single one of us, however, the greatly desired and envied suntan is a short-lived and temporary thing while the evil aftereffects are long-lasting and progressively more damaging. The sun's greatest power is sheer permanent damage to the skin.

Immediately, with overexposure, it can mean sunburn, blisters, cold sores, and other skin rashes and disturbances. In the longer term, over the years, it makes the skin sag before its time and promotes even in young people that dreaded enemy of youth—wrinkles. Along with the wrinkles comes a tough, leatherlike texture, crow's-feet around the eyes, permanent blotching and freckling, and deep crevices in the neck, the inner skin of the elbows, and other extra vulnerable areas.

As if that weren't bad enough, there is another horrifying result: skin cancer. Doctors have evidence that skin cancer brought on by too much sun is not confined to the aged; it can develop in persons under twenty years of age.

Remember, please, that the skin is a constantly overworked organ, ceaselessly replacing itself. The epidermis replaces itself completely about every twenty-eight days. Here's how it happens.

The cells in the deeper layer of the epidermis constantly divide into new cells and are pushed up to the outer layer.

They start to flake off when they reach the surface and are immediately replaced by fresh cells from below.

By the time the cells reach the surface, they have gone through a series of changes. From soft living cells, they have been changed to form a hard layer to act as the protective shell of the body. That "new" hard layer is really made up of about twenty closely woven layers covering the whole body surface in a melded protective coat.

Now add to this ceaseless task the burning of the ultraviolet rays of the sun. Think of the unreasonable strain on the skin and its normal job. It's no wonder that nature can do little to fight against the premature aging of the skin.

The strong light we receive from the sun is actually visible radiant energy. Among the sun's invisible waves of radiation are what we know as ultraviolet rays. It is those invisible rays that are responsible for your sunburn or your tan. It is those same rays that man is trying to capture to supply limitless energy for his everday needs. The potential of the sun's power is incredible. We've known for centuries that directly focusing the sun's rays on one spot can boil water and change it into steam. "Solar" stoves powered by ultraviolet rays have for decades cooked food and baked bread. We are working toward the day when pumps operated by solar energy will irrigate the desert and enable crops to grow in vast sections of the earth now suffering from food shortages.

Are you convinced yet of what the sun can do to make you look old—while you are still young? Its abuse is especially bad for the white race. White skin has a minimum of *melanin*, the brown coloring matter produced by cells called *melanoblasts* that lie just below the epidermis. The melanoblasts are activated by ultraviolet light and produce freckles and tanning in light skin. When the melanoblasts are assailed unceasingly by ultraviolet rays, along with the freckles and the tanning comes drying of the delicate underlayers of the skin and you get early wrinkling and sagging.

Now about vitamin D, which we all heard about in elementary grades. One important source of that vitamin, necessary to health and growth, we were told, was the sun. It was really important to development of the body. But the age groups to whom that was most vital—infants, toddlers, and small fry— rarely bake for hours in the sun on the beach or the front lawn. That's more the teenage thing.

Yet normally physical growth and development end during the late teens and early twenties. After that you can turn down the ultraviolet rays of the sun. The vitamin D that you get in your daily *balanced* diet, particularly in fortified milk, is enough.

For years sunlamps have enjoyed popularity as a way of holding on to a glamorous summer tan, particularly in those sections of the country with short sunny seasons. More recently "tanning booths" have rivaled sunlamps for public acceptance. Recognizing their potential danger, the federal government established regulations for tanning booths to guard against burns and eye injury; notice, however, that no warning is given against premature aging of the skin.

Skin specialists tell us, however, that natural and man-made ultraviolet light carry exactly the same danger.

Much advertising is currently devoted to over-the-counter drugs, creams, and lotions that provide sun screening. Supposedly they protect one from severe burning and encourage a swift and smooth tan. So good is business in that area that the manufacturers offer a wide variety of ingredients so that the gullible purchaser can choose products to fit individual needs.

The jury on the efficacy of those products is still out. It should be realized, however, that it is ultraviolet light that tans the skin. If that light is really screened out, there is no tanning. It should also be remembered that even a total sun screen won't work when it is washed off during swimming or sweated off in the baking sun.

So whether it's too much sun on the beach or exposure under a home sunlamp or in a tanning booth, it's all the same when it comes to premature aging of the skin and even the risk, now or later, of skin cancer.

Off Your Fanny—On Your Feet

Nourishment and exercise: two different guidelines for your life-style. But they're very much related, like two parts of a team that fights to the finish for your health, your good looks, your long life.

Nourishment and exercise are the stars of the team. The performance of one isn't much good without the other. The nourishing food we eat feeds the cells, the smallest units of which our bodies are composed; the physical activity of our bodies sparks or triggers the cells to help carry on all of life's activities.

Circulation

When push comes to shove, the whole deal is a matter of proper circulation of the blood through the body. The circulation is promoted mostly through the contraction and relaxation of the muscles, all over the body. When the circulatory system has its act together, it provides more food and oxygen to the cells and takes away waste materials more efficiently, thereby promoting their growth. All this is a special must for the teen and young adult years.

It's also important to keep the muscles in top shape. Even in children they can become flabby if they are seldom used or used improperly. Proper and regular exercise is the secret of keeping the muscles and joints in good condition.

The billions—some experts say over 100 trillion—of *cells* in your body don't sit around in separate slots like eggs in a carton. They're arranged in groups of certain types called *tissues*, to work together. Several tissues performing together like a chorus line make up an *organ*. Several organs (heart, blood vessels, lungs, liver, etc.) working together make up a *system* such as the cardiovascular system, in which the heart pumps blood through the blood vessels in circular action around and through the body.

Like all living things, animal or vegetable, the tissues constantly need a full supply of oxygen, whether the body is awake or asleep. That is the job of the lungs. The magic phrase you hear so often, "physical fitness," is the measurement of the ability of your heart and blood vessels and lungs to bring a suitable supply of oxygen to the tissues throughout your body.

You really wore out your mom when you were a toddler and started to walk; your dad no doubt described you as a perpetual energy machine, and much of your wild jumping and running around continued through the elementary school years. Instinctively, you were helping assure the supply of oxygen to your tissues. Nature was using that instinct to promote your growth and development.

Then with some of you, about the fifth or sixth grade, much of that physical activity came to a screeching halt. Partly that could be attributed to the routine of school years; imprisonment at a desk and more homework meant less time for it. Almost suddenly, it seemed, your body received a new set of signals and had to switch gears to slow down its physical activity.

At that time it's natural for you to start growing up, being quiet, sitting still when you should. But for your circulatory system, it's not too good to cancel out a lot of physical activity and exercise because you are still growing and developing.

Your complex cardiovascular system works on the principle of pressure/resistance, particularly in those years when it is essential to keep a balance between the two. No exercise, in spite of proper nutrition, no balance.

Maybe at your age your prime ambition isn't to live to be ninety or one hundred. That seems centuries away. If you're under eighteen years old, it probably never even occurs to you that someday you'll be what society calls "old."

But survival is our first instinct at any age, and no one really wants to die—certainly not prematurely. Don't take it from us. Every authority in the world will testify that a reasonable amount of exercise, every day throughout one's life, will help to extend the life span.

For young adults, predictions about a long life expectancy are taking on new meaning. What is "life expectancy"? The term refers to the average number of years that half or 50 percent of all persons alive in a particular year will survive. The figures are calculated annually by government agencies and insurance companies. In the mid-1980's the average life expectancy in the U.S. is about 74 years; it rises every few years.

If you're alive sixty or seventy years from now, you're just about guaranteed (barring accidents or like factors) that your senior years will be happier and healthier if you've kept up proper exercise habits.

The U.S. National Institute for Aging reported recently that if you are now twenty years of age or younger, those of you who will live past eighty-five will double among the population, as compared to today's figures, by the year 2020.

The Cheapie Walk

The nation now seems to be enjoying, or enduring, an unprecedented "physical fitness" craze. We see joggers in the streets in all kinds of weather the year round. Newspaper ads and TV commercials for exercise programs and gyms and salons are outnumbered only by that message directly to you and your group to buy designer jeans.

Even in ancient times physicians realized that walking was good for us. In more modern times, national meetings and conferences of experts have debated all forms of exercise, especially walking, and what it can do to help delay aging. Medical and physiology experts agree that walking is anybody's most efficient form of exercise and perhaps the only form of exercise that can be practiced safely and without strain all the days of one's life.

Regular walking, at any age, builds up the body's reserve of vitality and helps it battle stress. Walking keeps the leg bones nourished with enough mineral substances so that they are less likely to be injured or broken in an accident.

Hippocrates, the Greek father of medicine, said more than 2,000 years ago: "Walking is man's best medicine."

Walk, to and from high school, the local hangout, the movies, the pizza parlor. You certainly don't need special expensive threads; all it takes are comfortable clothes and a good, supporting pair of shoes.

Walking helps breathing, improves the appetite, helps to control weight. It also is of enormous benefit to—necessary for—a good cardiovascular system.

Let's see what happens to your body when you walk. For openers, all the muscles of the legs and feet get a good workout as they are forced to contract and relax with a consistent rhythm. The muscular action of the legs makes for a sort of twin pump with the heart muscle to get the blood circulating through the cardiovascular system.

As you know, fresh oxygenated blood, filled with "new" air, is pumped into the legs, as well as the rest of the body, through the arteries. The "used" blood with its impurities is pumped back through the veins, against the current, to the heart to be purified. Sometimes the blood doesn't move as fast as it should in the veins, and your legs feel tired and uncomfortable. Muscle activity in the legs gives that added push to pump the blood back to the heart and relieve the volume in the veins of the legs and the feet.

That improved circulation brings more food and oxygen to the cells, helps to remove wastes from the cells, and promotes their repair and the growth of new cells. Regular, vigorous walking can also keep all the leg and foot muscles, as well as the tendons, ligaments, and joints, in top condition.

Multiple Moves and Movement

Walking is a simple basic exercise, but not the only one. According to national estimates, there are currently 10 million Americans who jog, 15 million regular swimmers, 25 million cyclists, and close to 30 million serious tennis players among our population, of all ages. Americans are getting smarter: Based on recent polls, the number who work out in some form of exercise has about doubled in the last fifteen years or so—from 24 to 47 percent.

These statistics make cardiovascular specialists and cardiologists happy because they believe that regular exercise may well be an important part of the campaign to reduce the toll of America's top disease killer, coronary heart disease.

In recent years special types of exercises have been developed for adults and young adults. Chances are that you'll be hearing more and more about the four general types:

Aerobic exercises, which are the most strenuous, are designed to improve the organs and systems that are responsible for the body's use of oxygen—the heart, the lungs, and the blood vessels. They include jogging, running, bicycling, and swimming, activities that give a boost to your lungs to process more and purer air without too much involuntary effort on the part of the body's processes or routine. This strengthens the heart muscles and improves endurance. The secret of "aerobic activity" is continuous exercise, without rest in between; it is called "long slow distance activity."

Anaerobic exercise is of short and intense duration, followed by a period of rest. Examples are short games of handball or tennis and sprinting, which make a sudden and strong demand on heart and lungs and their activities.

Isometrics is a kind of nonexercise intended to build the body's strength without any actual movement. An isometric activity is best described as the contraction of a muscle or group of muscles against one another or against a hard, stationary object. An example is pushing hard against a wall. Isometrics are usually performed in 10- to 15-second time frames with the greatest possible effort. But there's a caution: Isometrics done to extremes can cause dizziness and fainting. The system failed to gain approval from the President's Council on Physical Fitness and Sports.

Isotonics covers what many of you will recognize as "pumping iron." It includes weight-lifting, push-ups, sit-ups, pull-ups, and a variety of other related exercises. Besides building and maintaining muscle mass, isotonics improves posture.

There you have it. Choose your own form of exercise and exercise program if you get serious about it. But remember, it should be regular. Set aside the time, every day, that you will devote to your exercise program. Sure, some kinds require costly exercise equipment, but maybe the investment will persuade you to keep it up and so get your money's worth.

Nevertheless, remember that simple walking is one of the best forms of exercise, open to everyone, especially good for your age, and requiring no fancy training or equipment. Some authorities say that, regardless of age, a person can stay fit by walking briskly about 20 miles a week, about three miles a day. And climb the stairs; don't take the elevator or escalator. You'll feel better, and you'll look better.

Warmup and Conditioning Exercises*

Walking is good exercise for the legs, heart and lungs, but it is not a complete exercise program. Persons who limit themselves to walking tend to become stiff and inflexible, with short, tight muscles in the back and the backs of the legs.

They also may lack muscle tone and strength in the trunk and upper body. These conditions can lead to poor posture and chronic lower-back pain, a problem that partially cripples or disables thousands of middle-aged and older Americans.

The exercises that follow are designed to increase flexibility and strength and to serve as a "warmup" for walking. Always do the exercises before walking.

Stretcher   Stand facing wall an arm's length away. Lean forward and place palms of hands flat against wall, slightly below shoulder height. Keep back straight, heels firmly on floor, and slowly bend elbows until forehead touches wall. Tuck hips toward wall and hold position for 20 seconds. *Repeat exercise with knees slightly flexed.*

Knee Pull   Lie flat on back with legs extended and arms at side. Lock arms around legs just below knees and pull knees to chest, raising buttocks slightly off floor. Hold for 10 to 15 counts. (If you have knee problems, you may find it easier to lock arms behind knees.) *Repeat exercise 3 to 5 times.*

Reach and Bend   Stand erect with feet shoulder-width apart and arms extended over head. Reach as high as possible while keeping heels on floor and hold for 10 counts. Flex knees slightly and bend slowly at waist, touching floor between feet with fingers. Hold for 10 counts. (If you can't touch the floor, try to touch the tops of your shoes.) *Repeat entire sequence 2 to 5 times.*

Situp   Several versions of the situp are listed in reverse order of difficulty (easiest one listed first, most difficult one last). Start with the situp that you can do three times without undue strain. When you are able to do 10 repetitions of the exercise without great difficulty, move on to a more difficult version.

1. Lie flat on back with arms at sides, palms down, and knees slightly bent. Curl head forward until you can see past feet, hold for three seconds, then lower to starting position. *Repeat exercise 3 to 10 times.*

2. Lie flat on back with arms at sides, palms down, and

knees slightly bent. Roll forward until upper body is at 45-degree angle to floor, then return to starting position. *Repeat exercise 3 to 10 times.*

3. Lie flat on back with arms at sides, palms down, and knees slightly bent. Roll foward to sitting position, then return to starting position. *Repeat exercise 3 to 10 times.*

4. Lie flat on back with arms crossed on chest and knees slightly bent. Roll forward to sitting position, then return to starting position. *Repeat exercise 3 to 10 times.*

5. Lie flat on back with hands laced in back of head and knees slightly bent. Roll forward to sitting position, then return to starting position. *Repeat exercise 3 to 15 times.*

---

*SOURCE: *Put Some Pep In Your Step.* Reprinted with permission from the President's Council on Physical Fitness and Sports.

Dope: High, Wide and (not so) Handsome

"Only a real dope touches dope," a public service ad said in a recent warning to young people.

Ironically, in generations past, the accusation that a teen-ager or a young adult was a "dope" was merely fighting words; it implied that he or she was not too bright, not with it, didn't have both oars in the water, wasn't playing with a full deck.

Sadly, today's "dope" among the young is a junkie, an addict, someone hung up on uppers, downers, highs, lows, marijuana, angel dust, or some such poison. One real horror in the picture is the fact that such addiction is no longer confined to the young of inner-city and poverty areas but is rampant in many high schools around the country, public and private, urban and rural.

What is a sad sermon on dope addiction and drug abuse doing in a book on nutrition for today's young people? It should be plain. It means that the one who uses drugs is not only canceling out the benefits of decent nourishment but also opting for bad health and black times, not only in adult years, but *now*. Dope can be quicker in ruining one's life and future than almost any other habit that might be named.

Older people as well as young adults are offenders. Pot parties have meant serious health hazards. Along with drivers drunk on alcohol, drug abusers form the greatest percentage of highway injuries and fatalities.

Statisticians say that almost every child or teenager will "experiment" with a drug, at least once. Not all will become addicts, by a long shot, but enough will do so and thereby queer all their career plans.

Drug addiction, which is usually launched in the early or late teen years with one experiment or experience, is not a "sin" or a moral abnormality; it's a disease. The young person often sees it as a cop-out to help in coping with day-to-day negatives or a quick fix for "really feeling good" without the tiresome efforts to work things out in the traditional way.

First of all, the young addict could never be in the running for a beauty contest. He or she becomes a slob in personal grooming, skeletonlike because of nourishment deprivation, lethargic or hyperactive, often with blotchy or spotty skin and chronically red and swollen eyes.

So-called illegal drugs and their abuse were not a lightning discovery of the late twentieth century. We have scientific testimony that their popularity dates back to ancient Egyptian and even prehistoric cultures. Many peoples have used some sort of drug as part of their life-style—chewing it, smoking it, or ingesting it as a pain-killer, as an aphrodisiac to spark sexual desire, or even as a miraculous "cure" for certain illnesses.

It was perhaps the unbelievable widespread use of marijuana in high schools, which surfaced explosively in the 1960's and 70's, that spotlighted the modern drug-addiction scene.

Several types of drugs, historical and traditional as well as recently developed, are in current use.

Those favored by teens and young adults are of three main types or classes: stimulants (substances that speed up activity) such as the amphetamines; depressants (downers) such as tranquilizers; and the psychedelics (mind expanders) such as marijuana, peyote, and the infamous LSD.

At this writing, the "in" thing is a lethal combination called

"T's and Blue's," a drug with the brand name Talwin and pentazerine, which can produce a quick high; doctors find it also brings on extreme euphoria or exaggerated sense of well-being, aggression, paranoia or feelings of persecution, hallucinations, and severe convulsions. Worse, infants born to mothers who are addicted to it often have too few fingers and toes, suffer from diarrhea and dehydration, and are in serious danger of infant death.

One reason for the popularity of T's and Blue's is that the combination is less expensive than other drugs, but actually they are all costly bummers. The "habit" costs the average user a minimum of $125 to $250 daily. The user who is hooked on any drug has to get the bread somewhere. Boys go in for robbery, mugging, burglary; young girls, too often into prostitution.

Young people of minority groups understandably get hooked on a type accessible to thin billfolds and slim budgets. Those of the so-called white middle class go more for the psychedelics, with marijuana and LSD top favorites. A twisted kind of caste system exists among dope users and addicts.

Observers believe that drug addiction, particularly among the young, may persist or even get worse. Despite the fact that drugs are illegal, it has become increasingly easy to obtain them. It has become easier for the teenager to make the "difficult transition" to young adulthood with the "sure-fire boosts" of drug use.

The terms "peer acceptance" and "peer pressure" are familiar but often get fuzzy in the way they are used. What do they mean? Simply, both mean what young people perceive as the acceptance or rejection of our ideas and hopes, what others in our age group think about what we do or don't do.

Adults often feel that if *we* "accept" our children in varying age groups for what they are and what they do, all is well for them. Nothing could be further from the truth. What really matters to the young is the sincere acceptance of *their* age

group, their own peers. This has been true from time imme-
morial; it is the increasing recognition of the fact that's new.
The young adult, in most cases, *has to have* friends and
acquaintances of the same or similar age group.

Seeking to satisfy the desire to be a swinging member of the
group, unfortunately it's only another step to the great adven-
ture of drugs—which among other new experiences holds out
a strange form of security against anxiety.

Regrettably, some reader may have already started down
the path of drug addiction, hooked on the popular and prolif-
erating pot even in the early teens. Dr. Jason Baron, Medical
Director of Deer Park Hospital, Deer Park, Texas, writing in
a recent issue of *Family Circle* magazine, points out:

> "During the last three years, the starting age for marijuana
> use has steadily decreased. Today in many middle- and
> upper-income communities, eleven is the *average* starting
> age. And national surveys clearly show that the younger a
> child starts pot, the more likely he is to get involved with
> other drugs. . . .

There is an ongoing controversy as to whether or not
marijuana—the sought-after smoke of teen and young-adult
experimenters—is harmless. Up to this point in time, the hard
and scientific evidence gives a loud and clear "No" to the
possibility of its harmlessness. Dr. Baron also points out that
moderate to heavy use of pot can damage the lungs, alter the
structure of brain cells, and impair sex and reproductive
functions.

Calling the use of marijuana the opening of a "real Pando-
ra's box" of negative results and complications, he continues:

> "Proponents of pot insist that it does not lead to the use of
> other, more dangerous drugs. Perhaps. But there are
> alarming indications that it does. For example, among the
> 50 percent of high-school seniors who smoke marijuana, 43

percent use one or more illegal drugs. Among youngsters who don't smoke pot, the use of other drugs is almost unknown."

You'd like to think straight when you are in hot or secret pursuit of that cute sophomore or senior class president. And a decent report card might bring permission and blessing to stay out a little later at night.

Here's the monkey wrench that can be thrown into your hopes and plans. Marijuana, without the shadow of a doubt, will impair your thinking, your learning, your ability to get your driver's license. As a pot smoker, you might be invited to a pot party, but you'll never get that scholarship for college, or the use of the family car—because chances are you'll never pass the driver's test.

Need more evidence? The National Institute of Drug Abuse has put the hex on marijuana and its use as a "major and serious health hazard."

Your brain has gone through a surge of growth and development during the early and later teen years. It's had enough to cope with. Don't blow it all with an unhappy trip, shot off the launching pad with a few joints of pot.

While the jury is still out, with the likelihood that it will return a definite verdict of "guilty of premeditated murder" for the defendant called by any drug name, DON'T! Maybe it's a hot item with your peers right now. But it's not cool. As a matter of fact, it's real dumb.

The Cigarette and the Cardiovascular System

According to at least one federal official, there's a form of smoking that's just about as bad for all of us as the marijuana weed.

Every pack of cigarettes sold in the United States carries these words on the side: "Warning: The Surgeon General Has Determined That Cigarette Smoking Is Dangerous to Your

Health." It's meant to try to reach adults who smoke and to offer some preventive medicine to young nonsmokers.

But more teenagers are smoking these days, we're told, and they're starting earlier. And something has been added: a difference in trends between the sexes. Your dad and grand-dad and uncle may be among the wise owls who have given up smoking. Not so, and not so good, for the females. Some of you have moms or aunts or sisters who still light up in spite of the warnings.

Meanwhile, cigarette prices continue to soar. The government constantly raises taxes on certain items that are most definitely detrimental to health. "Human nature" being what it is, people will drink and smoke, and the government turns that fact to its advantage.

A national survey has revealed that while smoking among teens and young adults has dropped about 25 percent since 1974, for the first time more girls than boys in those age groups are now smoking. But, it is predicted, a boy who takes up smoking before age fifteen, and continues to smoke, is only half as likely to live to age seventy-five as a boy who never smokes.

A high percentage of doctors, psychologists, and behavioral scientists believe that it's not entirely the young people's fault. On the carpet are their parents and teachers who have failed to help them fully understand that "the weed" and "the sauce" are *drugs*—habit-forming and addictive, dangerous, life-threatening and life-shortening.

Today's American young people are said to be on the whole brighter, more responsive, and generally more intelligent than those of previous generations. So why do so many of them ignore the antismoking warnings, widespread publicity, and outright campaigns against the killers?

Back between 1950 and 1960, proof positive was already available that smoking is a direct hit-man for lung cancer and a sure-fire risk factor for chronic bronchitis, emphysema, coronary heart disease, and a host of other nasties that make life (if it continues) the very dregs.

No case is made for Uncle Stogie's smelly black cigar or great-grandma's ugly clay pipe. No detailed research was done on either. It's the three-inch cigarette that science has proved a real killer.

Yet tobacco *is* the cigarette, right? We could ask why we don't start earlier to teach our kids that tobacco and the nicotine that it contains lead to addiction. First we must help them to understand that "addiction," considered an adult problem, can begin in very early years.

What do we mean by "addiction"? Basically, it is the compulsive or obsessive use of a destructive drug over which the user has no voluntary control.

Think about what goes into a cigarette: some harmless white or brown paper rolled around some dried weeds. Let's see what really happens when we flick our Bic at the end of that neat cigarette cylinder.

As the cigarette is lit, the lungs inhale the smoke that lighting produces and then send the lethal contents of the tobacco throughout the body via the arteries and veins. The two main poisons contained in tobacco smoke are nicotine and carbon monoxide.

Nicotine is a poisonous alkaloid that is colorless, complex, and bitter, the chief active principle of tobacco. It is sometimes used in insecticides.

Carbon monoxide is a waste product that is also found in the exhaust fumes of automobiles. In cigarette smoke it competes with oxygen to combine with hemoglobin, the vital component of the red blood cells. Once in combination, the two stick together like glue. The hemoglobin is able to carry either oxygen or carbon monoxide; it cannot carry both. The carbon monoxide wins out, and the body is short-changed of the oxygen needed to nourish it.

That's not all. The nicotine in the cigarette constricts (squeezes and narrows) the veins and slows the blood flow to the limbs, the brain, and the body.

"Try it, you'll like it" isn't the story with your first cigarette or two. Right off, you'll probably hate the heat and the bad taste and bitterness it leaves in your mouth. But you can get used to it, if you're bent on that form of suicide. The experts tells us that peer pressure and the flaky notion that smoking is "sophisticated" defeat the unpleasant taste, and now we may have another stupid nicotine addict.

Smoking won't make you beautiful or handsome or popular. Here's what it *will* do. The smoke will get in your eyes and make them red and veiny. Your fingertips will take on an ugly brown and smell nasty. Your breath and your clothes will smell awful. And your wind will be gone but not forgotten as you suddenly realize that—since you started to smoke—your running time, swimming distance, or endurance on the ballfield or the tennis court is cut to ribbons.

Maybe a friend told you that cigarettes will help you lose weight. Maybe. But if that happens, it's mostly because the poisons that cling to your teeth and mouth after smoking make everything, even junk food, taste terrible. So you eat less because you enjoy almost nothing. Nice job of robbing your body of true nourishment and nutrients for the iffy possibility that you *might*, much later on, fit into a smaller size dress or pair of slacks.

If you resist the temptation, think of what you'll save. Money, lots of it. Brown fingertips and yellow teeth. Cigarette burns on your fingers or your lips. Little holes in your favorite clothes from a live ash dropped from a cigarette. Lungs tinted a sinister brown-black.

Demon Rum Gets a D

Why do we square adults get so uptight about the idea that alcohol might get the drop on high schoolers and young adults? For the most part it's because we know that, in terms of chronological age, you're just not ready to handle it.

There's evidence for that conclusion. Consider that most drunk driving and even highway deaths show an unsteady teenager, usually a boy, as the prime offender? Incomplete growth and development and lack of driving experience make a questionable combination. Add liquor to that, and we've got serious trouble.

It is for several good reasons that alcohol is classed with drugs and narcotics. They all cloud your judgment and reactions, destroy your mental and physical coordination, and, for closers rather than openers, often make you pass out. Although it is known as a depressant, alcohol means different strokes for different folks. It has a wide pattern of negative effects. The drinking bout has a cycle; depending on amounts and types, it can stimulate as well as depress, give a real "dope high" as well as tranquilize.

If you're about to tap a six-pack or have already gotten into your parents' liquor cabinet, you're in no mood to analyze chemical content, yours or the alcohol's. Instead, you've been kidding yourself that it made you feel good, less shy, more comfortable in the company of friends and associates.

Let's see what really happens with the alcoholic drink.

Your body absorbs alcohol, first and immediately, in both the stomach and the small intestine. It can show up right away on your breath and as soon as five minutes in your blood: two reasons why the police can make those reliable tests on suspects they pick up.

Alcohol is then transported by the bloodstream to various parts of the body, the spinal fluid, the urine, and the pulmonary (lung) air sacs. The alcohol is then changed by oxidation into carbon monoxide, a small percentage of which is shed by the body chemically, in an unchanged state, in urine, perspiration, and respiration.

The main site of metabolism for alcohol is the liver. Alcohol is changed by the liver into *acetaldehyde* (a colorless, volatile, water-soluble liquid), partly by the processes of the "oxidase system," dehydrating the body as it mixes with oxygen.

We need to talk here about what happens when alcohol and drugs are taken together. Alcohol can stimulate and speed up the action of barbiturates and sedatives. It is believed that this may explain why the combined action of alcohol and sedatives in the brain can in extreme cases cause death. Further research on this may change some verdicts of "suicide" to "accidental death," caused by ignorance of what can happen when a drug is "washed down" with scotch or even beer or wine.

On the other hand, alcohol taken with other drugs can interfere with metabolism of the drug. Researchers believe that alcohol competes with the other drug for the enzymes, or assistants to the body's chemical processes and changes, that are necessary to each of them.

Even a small excursion into alcohol, particularly in the young adult years, can wreck the ability of the intestines to absorb such nutrients as glucose, calcium, amino acids, vitamin B-12, and folic acid, all essentials to healthy blood building. This is an important part of the reason why malnutrition and "borderline anemia" are sometimes traced to heavy drinking or alcoholism.

The basic problem, of course, is that alcoholic intake has the power to counteract the body's natural desire for good food and a balanced diet. The drinker substitutes the "empty calories" of liquor for the nourishing calories of food.

Certainly alcohol attacks the liver, the blood circulation, and the brain centers with a vengeance. But another victim of attack is the hard-working heart. Alcohol takes direct action on the strain causing irregulation of the heart muscle; it can bring on elevation in cardiac rate and output. So it can raise the blood pressure, weaken the heart muscle by starving it of nutrition, and—going on to other parts of the body—even damage skeleton muscle and muscle fiber.

So in both the long and the short run, this form of addictive narcotic—alcohol—is bad news. Add up what it can do to shaft your morale: fuzz up your school work, take the edge off your appetite, make you feel tired all the time, give you the look of an unmade bed. If you're smart, you'll keep to soft drinks. If you're brilliant, you'll turn to water and fruit juice when you need a drink.

CHAPTER • XVI

Planning Ahead: Life Span and Today's Menu

Sure, you're pretty young to worry about this. But you're not too young to plan for it, right now!

If you're anywhere from twelve to eighteen years old, you may have another sixty or more years to go, barring accidental death or a premature fatal illness.

The fact is that under normal circumstances, you'll be living a lot longer than your grandparents did—even than your parents and uncles and aunts.

Life expectancy, the average length of life for the population, could be 80 years by 1990. Since the turn of the century, the average of life expectation has gone from 47.3 in 1900 to almost 74 years today. At that rate, and at the same rate of progress, average life expectancy could reach 100 by the turn of the century.

The U.S. Census Bureau estimates that the elderly population will be over 32 million in the year 2000. The American Association for the Advancement of Science estimates that the figure will be closer to 36 million. The Association also predicts that life expectancy figures will continue to rise into the twenty-first century and will reach about 95 years early in the new century.

The question is, how are we going to use those extra years. Will most of us, the future "elderly" (over sixty-five years of age), need artificial aids such as canes, walkers, or wheelchairs to get around? Why do some people we know look and act "old" when their birthdays total thirty or forty? Why do others seem to stay young and vigorous at seventy or eighty?

Turned Tables

Right now, the hopes and dreams and the future of the economy are on you, the young adult. Advertisements on style, on clothes, on music—you name it—are directed toward the young. There's money in it for them, the merchandisers feel, if they cater to you and your buying habits.

The tables will soon turn, if we know our Madison Avenue. The greater part of the population with the money to spend, in this country and in others, is growing older. The time will come when there are many more people over sixty-five than under to buy goods.

How are we going to be able to use these precious extra years? How are we going to cope with the prospect that hopes for the fountain of youth give way to a half-century of painful degeneration?

At this writing, prospects are dim. Increasingly, people are dying of illness associated with old age. It is estimated that 75 percent of all deaths among people over sixty-five are from the terrible trio of heart disease, cancer, and stroke.

Medical leaders have faced the prospect squarely and are beginning to concentrate on *gerontology*, the science of aging and the problems of the aged.

The National Institute of Aging since 1974 has been part of the National Institutes of Health. Every sizable university and medical school in the country has an Institute on Aging. For the first time, medical schools are seeking to turn out young physicians interested medically and scientifically in older people.

We must change life-styles, physically and psychologically,

if we want to make the best use of those later years of life.
Our genes, those heriditary factors present in our cells, will
continue to influence how long we live. Geographic factors of
where we live will always have a bearing on our individual life
span.

But as scientists intensify their study of aging, more and
more zero in on nutrition and how it has affected each stage
of life as we've gone along. They argue that there is a close
connection between the eating habits of early and youthful
years and the onset and severity of the so-called degenerative
diseases.

Nutrition and Long Life

To emphasize that there must be a real relationship
between longevity and nutritional health over the years, let's
review the basics, once again.

Every one of the trillions of living cells in the human body
(not a few or a selective percentage) has to have its *daily* share
of nutrients to do its specific life-sustaining work. If even a
small number of cells don't get the means of doing their work,
the entire body suffers because the cells are so dependent on
one another.

The experts believe now that even a brief nutritional short-
changing of a very few cells launches the early stages of the
physical aging process.

Remember that the red blood cells, which carry hemoglobin, transport the oxygen that sparks the working of the
rest of the body. When the tissues that produce the red cells
are undernourished, too few of the cells are made. If the
nutrients supplied are of an inferior grade, *anemia*—lack of
vitality due to a shortage of red blood cells—can result.

The signals or symptoms of this anemia are themselves
characteristic of aging: a bad or sallow color of the face, a
lack of ease in breathing, indigestion, poor appetite, dizziness.
These aging characteristics can also very well be the beginning
signs of a breakdown in health.

If poor nutrition can mean a blow to healthy and zestful life, the opposite is true to all intents and purposes. Good nutrition, at any age and particularly in young adulthood, can offer a healthy plus to the current quality of life and perhaps a postponement by years of the ravages of age.

Neat Nutrition for Nineteen or Ninety

The bottom line is that sound nutrition is not only smart for all age groups: Without it, nothing else really matters and nothing is accomplished in the way of pep, production, or popularity. No engine has been invented that will perform well on inferior or inadequate fuel.

It is basic that the human being needs a diet of well-balanced foods even before he or she is born—in the mother's womb, fed as a fetus through her placenta. That must continue, and even improve in content and balance, as the child is born and eats on its own, giving it a decent start in physiological life and development.

The family car carries no lifetime guarantee; some cynics say that today's "built-in obsolescence" means your dad's lucky if his car lasts two years. Your body is the only engine to have a lifetime guarantee, but there's a catch. It's largely up to you to decide the length of that guarantee. How long you live, and how well you live through a long life, depend largely on how you treat your body—and feed it.

"You are what you eat," no doubt about it. We know that overweight and underweight, scraggly hair, unhealthy skin, bad teeth, poor performance in school or on the athletic field are in large part due to faulty or inadequate diet.

Join the club: the club of young adults who are demanding the facts of sound nutrition and following the guidelines. Inflation is having a lot to do with the scene. Parents who find a trip to the supermarket a progressive financial shock are or should be sick and tired of additives, synthetics, fillers. They want nutrition for those high prices. Back them up!

You're still young and have time to get food-smart, more

time than do your parents and teachers.

How much time and happiness you can map out on your personal chart depends on what you do with that knowledge. Mind your menus. Good luck, and long life.

A Humorist Looks at Nutrition

It's an educated guess that you have already learned that things are constantly changing in this life, too much, too soon. That moan-and-groan isn't only a complaint of senior citizens. You guys and dolls, into designer jeans and shirts, know how both styles and prices change, it seems almost monthly. What about the doubled deductions in your parents' checkbook after writing a new check for your tuition?

One thing doesn't change much, however: good old-fashioned American humor. Today's standup comics look a little different (get paid a lot more), but much of their material—with a few (X-rated) changes in language—was lifted in essence from the comic routines of decades and even generations ago.

We meant this book to be deadly serious. After all, we aim to help you live a healthful young adult life and to extend your life span with the best quality as well as quantity in years. However, we also hoped to come down with not too heavy a scene.

So we have concluded with a little comic relief from the late, great humorist Robert Charles Benchley (1889–1945). Benchley knew a little about physiology and that branch of it dealing with metabolism and growth, and he used that carefree knowledge to tickle his literary funnybone.*

*From *Inside Benchley* by Robert Benchley, "The Romance of Digestion," "Cell-formations and Their Work," copyright 1925 by Harper & Row, Publishers, Inc.; renewed 1953 by Gertrude D. Benchley, reprinted by permission of Harper & Row Publishers, Inc.

Cell-formations and Their Work

It is only recently that science has found out the exact structure of the tiny cell-formations which go to make up life. Only yesterday, in fact.

Every higher animal starts life as a single cell. This much is obvious. Look at the rainbow. Look at the formation of frost on the window-pane. Don't look now. Wait a minute... Now look.

This cell measures no more than 1/125 of an inch in diameter at first, but you mustn't be discouraged. It looks like nothing at all, even under the strongest microscope, and before we knew just how important they were, they were often thrown away. We now know that if it were not for these tiny, tiny cells, we should none of us be here today. This may or may not be a recommendation for the cells. *Quien sabe?*

Shortly after the cell decides to go ahead with the thing, it gets lonely and divides itself up into three similar cells, just for company's sake and to have someone to talk to. They soon find out that they aren't particularly congenial, so they keep on dividing themselves up into other cells until there is a regular mob of them. Then they elect an entertainment committee and give a show.

After the show, there is a fight, and the thing breaks up into different cliques or groups. One group think they are white corpuscles or *phagocytes*. Others go around saying that they are *red* corpuscles and to hell with the white.

The other groups of cells devote themselves to music, aesthetic dancing, and the formation of starch which goes into dress-shirts. They are all very happy and very busy, and it's nobody's business *what* they do when they aren't working. We certainly are not going to snoop into that here.

We must take up, however, the work of the brain-cells, as it is in the brain that the average man of today does his thinking. (Aha-ha-ha-ha-ha-ha!)

Oh, let's *not* take up the brain-cells. You know as much

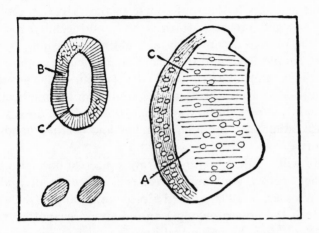

Differentiation of cells in the lens of an eye. Doesn't mean a thing

about them as anybody does, and what's the use anyway? Suppose you *do* learn something today. You're likely to die tomorrow, and there you are.

And we *must* go into the question of the size of these cells. That really is important. In about 1/150000 of a cubic inch of blood there are some five million cells afloat. This is, as you will see, about the population of the City of London, except that the cells don't wear any hats. Thus, in our whole body, there are perhaps (six times seven is forty-two, five times eight is forty, put down naught and carry your four, eight times nine is seventy-two and four is seventy-six, put down six and carry your seven and then, adding, six, four, three, one, six, naught, naught, naught), oh, about a billion or so of these red corpuscles alone, not counting overhead and breakage. In the course of time, that runs into figures.

Now when it comes to reproduction, you have to look out. In the cuttlefish, for example, there is what is known as "gree-sion" or budding. The organism as a whole remains unaltered, except that one small portion of it breaks off and goes into business for itself. This, of course, makes a very pretty picture, but gets nowhere. In the case of multicellular animals, like the orange, it results in a frightful confusion.

We should have said that there are two classes of animals, unicellular and multicellular. From the unicellular group we get our coal, iron, wheat and ice, and from the multicellular our salt, pepper, chutney and that beautiful silk dress which milady wears so proudly. Woolen and leather goods we import.

You will see then that by grafting a piece of one species on another species, you can mix the cells and have all kinds of fun. Winkler, in 1902, grafted a piece of Solanum (the genus to which the potato belongs) onto a stock of another kind, and then, after the union had been established, cut the stem across, just at the point of junction. The bud was formed of the intermingled tissues of the two species and was most peculiar-looking.

Winkler was arrested.

The Romance of Digestion

When you take a bite of that delicious cookie, or swallow a morsel of that nourishing bread, do you stop to think of the marvelous and intricate process by means of which Mother Nature is going to convert it into bone and sinew and roses for those pretty cheeks? Probably not, and it is just as well. For if you did stop to think of it at that time, you would unquestionably not be able to digest that cookie—or that nourishing bread.

But whether you think of it or not this exciting process of digestion is going on, day in and day out, sometimes pretty badly but always with a great show of efficiency. It is, on the whole, probably one of the worst-done jobs in the world.

First you must know that those hard, white edges of bone which you must have noticed hundreds of times along the

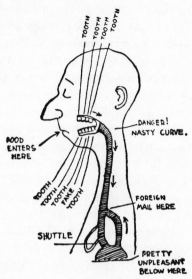

Cross section of human food duct, showing ludicrous process of self-styled "Digestion"

front of your mouth, are "teeth," and are put there for a very definite purpose. They are the ivory gates to the body. They are Nature's tiny sentinels, and if you have ever bitten yourself, you will know how sharp they can be, and what efficient little watchmen they are. Just you try to slip your finger into your mouth without your teeth's permission, and see how far you get. Or try to get it out, once they have captured it.

Now these thousands of brave little soldiers, the teeth, which we have in our mouths, take the food as it comes through the air (in case you are snapping at a butterfly) or from the fork, and separate it into its component parts (air, land, and water). In this process, the teeth are aided by the tongue, which is that awful-looking thing right back of your teeth. Don't look at it!

The tongue (which we may call the escalator of the mouth or Nature's nobleman for short), and the teeth toss the food back and forth between them until there is nothing left of it, except the little bones which you have to take out between your thumb and forefinger and lay on your butter-plate. In doing this be careful that the bone is really on the butter-plate and that it does not stick to your finger so that you put it back into your mouth again on the next trip, for this would make the little white sentries very angry and they might all drop out.

And now comes the really wonderful part of the romance which is being enacted right there under your very eyes. A chemical reaction on the tongue presses a little button which telegraphs down, down, down, 'way down to the cross old Stomach and says: "Please, sir, do you want this food or don't you?" And the Stomach, whom we shall call "Prince Charming" from now on, telegraphs (or more likely writes) back: "Yes, dear!" or "You can do what you like with it for all of me." Just as he happens to feel at the time.

And then, such a hurry and bustle as goes on in the mouth! "Foodie's going to visit Stomach!" all the little teeth cry, and rush about for all the world as if they were going themselves. "All aboard, all aboard!" calls out the tongue, and there is a great ringing of bells and blowing of whistles and bumping of porters and in the midst of it all, the remnants of that delicious cookie seated nervously on the tongue, ready to be taken down on its first journey alone, down to see Prince Charming. For all the joyousness of the occasion, it is a little sad, too. For that bit of cookie is going to get some terribly tough treatment before it is through.

The food is then placed on a conveyor, by means of which it is taken to the Drying Room, situated on the third floor, where it is taken apart and washed and dried, preparatory to going through the pressing machines. These pressing machines are operated by one man, who stands by the conveyor as it brings the food along and tosses it into the vats. Here all rocks and moss are drawn off by mechanical pickers and the food subjected to treatment in a solution of sulphite, a secret process which is jealously guarded. From here the food is taken to the Playroom where it plays around awhile with the other children until it is time for it to be folded by the girls in the bindery, packed into neat stacks, and wrapped for shipment in bundles of fifty. Some of these bundles, the proteins, are shipped to the bones of the body, others, the hydrates, go to making muscle, while a third class, the sophomores, contribute to making fatty tissue which nobody wants, that is, not if he has any pride at all about his appearance. The by-products are made into milk-bottle caps, emery wheels, and insurance calendars, and are sold at cost.

Thus we see how wonderfully Nature takes care of us and our little troubles, aided only by sodamint and bicarbonate.

This book may be kept

FOURTEEN DAYS

A fine will be charged for each day the book is kept overtime.

GAYLORD 142

PRINTED IN U.S.A.